Realities Of A Stroke

THE GOOD, THE BAD, AND THE TRUTH

Cleothus Bell

Realities of A Stroke Copyright © 2011 Cleothus Bell

DISCLAIMER:
Information in this book is provided for informational purposes only and is not intended as medical advice nor is it intended to replace a medical doctor. You should not use the information contained herein for diagnosing or treating any health problem. If you have, or suspect that you have, a medical problem, promptly contact your health care provider. Information and statements in this book regarding health has not been evaluated by the medical profession and is not intended to diagnose, treat, cure, or prevent any medical condition. All decisions regarding a person's care should be made by a doctor, a nurse or healthcare provider.

ISBN 978.0.578.08390.2
Library of Congress Control Number 2011905976

Printed in United States of America

BELLCLE Publishing
East St. Louis, IL

Realities Of A Stroke
THE GOOD, THE BAD, AND THE TRUTH

Table of Contents

Dedication

Acknowledgements

Preface

Chapter 1...Telling It Like It Is

Chapter 2 ....Showdown With Stroke #1

Chapter 3...........................Should've, Would've, Could've

Chapter 4............................... Showdown With Stroke #2

Chapter 5.. A Friend Within

Chapter 6...........Nine Months of Botox With No Results

Chapter 7.................................Back Home After Stroke #2

Chapter 8.................................Showdown With Stroke #3

Chapter 9..............................Back Home After Stroke #3

Chapter 10 ....Walk a Mile to Gain an Inch

Chapter 11 .... A Need to Know But Nowhere to Go

Chapter 12 .... Up Front and No Sugar Coating

Chapter 13.. About Strokes

Frequently Asked Questions

About the Author

Book Order Form

Dedication

This book is dedicated to my oldest son, Little Cle, who was killed five months before my last stroke. To my mother Pearl, who passed away one year after the last stroke. To my girlfriend, Kim, who has been by my side after all three strokes, no matter when, where or what; and to Kaden Bell, my big six-year old son, who makes it a joy to wake up every day.

Acknowledgements

To Cleo Harris, Kim's mother and my telephone buddy who passed away two months after my mother. To my sister, Lillie, who was with me almost every day at the rehabilitation institute and after I returned home. To my friend, Derrick Glover, for his assistance in my at home rehabilitation. A special thank you, to the therapists at St. Elizabeth Rehabilitation Center in Belleville Illinois, for their continuous dedication and support. To my cousin, Shelia E. (Bell) Lipsey, with her special skills and knowledge of writing, editing and formatting, made the completion of my book possible.

Preface

During my struggles to reclaim my life after the second stroke, I did not think about other people in my situation that may not have had the mental strength, fortitude or motivation needed to weather this storm. As years passed, many people approached me on different occasions and posed questions about my life after my stroke. They basically wanted to know how long I had been dealing with my stroke and how I managed to keep such a good spirit all this time.

Initially, I was caught off guard, because I did not realize how clear it was to others that my disability was the result of having had a stroke. I had not realized how much of an affect this type of illness had on the lives of others. I guess people were looking for answers but were limited on where to go and get them.

Their main question to me was *how did I cope with my situation?* After I talked with them they would mention a loved one at home who needed to hear my words. Sometimes these individuals were friends, but 99% of the time they were total strangers. I ran into concerned people many times and at many different places, for instance the mall, grocery stores, convenient stores, and sometimes while visiting someone at the hospital.

I heard many different stories of stroke survivors coming home after weeks and months of therapy and after having made lots of improvement with their disability and then giving up after being home for a while. To hear the same stories over and over and other stories with similarities by others was really unbelievable. I had focused so on getting my own disability under control that I never thought of the many people out there that just could not deal with their situation for whatever the reason. I did know that dealing with this disability day in and day out could get pretty tiresome and annoying, but my daily thought was that I wanted to do better.

Because of my disabilities, my everyday restrictions were enormous. Each day I had to look at the simple everyday tasks in life as being a struggle and a challenge. I had to face the normal daily routines as major challenges, but I would not accept spending the rest of my life struggling while trying to deal with these problems. I knew that having the physical and mental strength and staying consistent had always been the way to win or be successful in spite of obstacles. The more you work to better a difficult situation the easier the struggle will get, so my thoughts were instead of sitting around doing nothing why not spend my time and energy on trying to improve my situation.

My intentions originally were not to write a book but to prepare notes for a date schedule as a motivational speaker for stroke survivors. Well one thing led to another when I started to put pen and paper together, and while jotting down notes I began to realize that after my second stroke, a lot had happened in my life. I guess I was so focused and determined on getting a handle on my life I never took the time to think about the steps I took along the way.

There were adjustments made constantly which were very significant to the daily routine of my day to day living. My many accomplishments were met with faithful commitments, and by setting goals and putting forth the effort to meet them.

After the insurance had reached the limits of financing my therapy treatment, I still had a long way to go but I was still determined to get my life back to normal with or without the help of others. I had set out on a mission to improve my life and to never waver. Through the many obstacles along the way I simply went around them if I could not get over them, and I did not dwell on the things I could not do, but to get stronger and better at what I could do. My mission was to get as much as I could out of what I had to work with.

The stroke was my own personal war. A war that was very confusing. A war I had not prepared properly for. A battle so long, it seems as though it will never end. A war I brought home with far-reaching effects on my family. The stroke changed everything in my life. After becoming severely disabled I was given physical treatment to my body but there was no treatment for my thoughts and emotions. Something no one could predict was coming and with no prediction of an end. A situation I was not trained for, but eventually it trained me and my focus on life. It enabled me to see and feel the sufferings of others. It taught me to see, feel and reach out to the pain of others and not just my pain.

A word to you, the stroke victim, sufferer, survivor and person: I feel your pain. Not a painful pain but a pain of suffering. A pain that makes you want to scream out while you wonder if anyone will hear you or more importantly, feel you. Your intense sorrows are your pain, but know that you are not alone. A stroke can happen to anyone. It happened to me, and this is my story.

Chapter 1
Telling It Like It Is
The Good, the Bad and the Truth

To all stroke survivors, your caregivers, your families, and your friends, thank you for taking the time to read this book. *Realities of a Stroke* contains concepts about me, a three time stroke survivor, who felt a need to share feelings, emotions and experiences with you, some which are good, and some not so good. Above all else, I seek to give some measure of comfort and encouragement by relaying information to stroke survivors and the people involved in their lives.

My objective in putting my story into words is not to try to make you happy or sad, but hopefully to assist you in thinking about and understanding some of the circumstances that might happen that could play a significant role in your life during your recovery from a stroke.

Whether you are a stroke victim, a loved one, a family member or a friend, this is to increase your awareness about what happened, what could have happened, what can happen and what needs to happen and why.

In our own way, each stroke survivor is alone. We harbor a magnitude of emotions. Many of us have entered into the darkness of a stroke and did not return.

Sometimes, the difference between coming out or not coming out or not coming out as whole as we might have after having had a stroke, rests in the hands of others. I discovered that the future of a stroke survivor often lies in the hands of inexperienced decision makers, non-caring, impatient, neglectful, money savers, sleepy, work dodgers, overtime workers, and fraud seekers. Fortunately we are blessed with plenty of people who have remained dedicated and still genuinely care for us.

I am saying to you now, that I am extending the word as it is and without sugar coating what I have personally seen, heard and read. Stroke survivors, we are not on a vacation at the beach. This is a debilitating illness to the mind, to the body and to our livelihood. But you are not alone.

Each year, almost 740,000 Americans suffer a stroke, and more than 137,000 of those people die. But even for survivors, a stroke puts everything you know at risk: your identity, your skills, and your dreams.

Those of you who have survived a stroke should know how lucky, fortunate and blessed you are. You are needed for a larger cause. With the experience you received from your suffering and surviving such an ordeal, you have been chosen to pass on to others, your knowledge of recovery. You have been chosen because there are not enough experienced helpers in the world who can actually feel your pain.

My aim is to help elevate your awareness during your journey back. Despite the difficulties and setbacks you surely have experienced, your motivation, determination and perseverance can make a difference in your recovery.

During the onset of a stroke, you usually are unable to think clearly. Initially, you may not immediately realize the conditions that could possibly hinder or help your situation during your road to recovery. It is difficult to adjust immediately to the affects of this type of illness, especially during the first few weeks.

There were no seminars to prepare you for making immediate adjustments after having suffered a stroke. A stroke victim is hardly ever, if ever, prepared for the onset. I do not believe there has ever been a case when a stroke victim has gone to the hospital with their bags already packed and a note left at the house telling everyone what happened, where to go and what to do. A stroke can happen in a matter of seconds. It is sudden, quick, and in many cases, it leaves permanent damage. It can incapacitate you for the rest of your life. This is an illness that sometimes strikes with a mild, physical disorder, before the overwhelming experience of devastation strikes. It can also be accompanied suddenly by a full physical, disabling force at the beginning. Either way, you will not be prepared for the aftermath.

One of the conditions that may possibly come into play that you may not be aware of or think about at the beginning of a stroke, is the amount of pressure that can be placed on the hospital and rehabilitation institute, whether directly or indirectly by insurance providers. You probably will not realize that you are being evaluated for your future progress to determine the amount of treatment you will need, and/or will be granted before alternative steps are introduced. You may not understand the dire need for motivation and a good response to treatment in a short amount of time. Instead, a stroke survivor is trying to adjust to the illness and trying to figure out what happened, why it happened and at what point will things start to get better, and hoping someone can make things better as soon as possible.

At this critical stage in your life, your immediate

future is in the hands of the medical professionals assigned to your case, whether it is through inpatient or outpatient treatment. Hopefully, the medical professionals are still dedicated and have not lost the desire to put their patient's recovery first.

The medical professional, after treating dozens of patients per month, is quite possibly aware of the limited time allowed for treatment for a particular patient. They also know of the progress that's needed for that particular patient, but for some reason cannot or just simply is unable to express this valuable information to the patient or the patient's family early in the treatment process. The medical professionals in charge of the treatment should know when there is a need to motivate the patient. And if they personally cannot do it or does not have the time, then the task of locating a great motivator should not be that difficult. This can be another medical professional or another stroke survivor with a determined attitude. There have been stroke survivors released from the institute or presently in the facility who may be able to help. Sometimes just hearing words about progress from another stroke survivor can be inspiring enough to conjure up the determination needed for a stroke sufferer to get to the next level of their rehabilitation. This approach, if successful, could make the job much easier between the therapist and the patient.

I recall several mornings when speakers were brought in to the rehabilitation unit to talk to us in what I call a gathering of the wheelchairs. They spoke about healthcare, stroke conditions, and other related subjects. A stroke victim in a wheelchair, in the early stages of a stroke, with agonizing feelings affecting their mind, body and soul, is unable to feel any significant connection to most of, if not all, of what the speaker is saying. At least 99% of the time during these sessions patients are in such a bad way that they simply want to get back to bed.

To hear from another stroke survivor could possibly be a positive enough session to which a stroke victim could connect with. Another stroke person could possibly get and keep the attention of the stroke victims long enough for them to realize some of the important steps they need to take to begin their process of recovery. A stroke victim, at this time is feeling so alone and confused with many inner emotions about this illness. They have no recollection of the word hope and what it means at this time. Seeing another stroke person and hearing their words of encouragement at this early stage of their illness could be an important missing link to putting some sense of hope into their everyday thoughts.

During a couple of sessions I wanted to say out loud to the speaker that no one was listening. I knew first hand why they were unable to listen, because if anyone felt half as bad as I did, then no one understood anything that was being said and even more so, could care less. The many agonizing feelings going through a stroke sufferer's body at this stage can only be felt by another stroke victim. Knowing this, I wanted to talk to the stroke persons in the room. I felt the need to communicate but I would have needed a push from someone. If I knew that someone wanted a stroke survivor to share their feelings of hope to other stroke survivors, then despite how bad I was feeling I would have been the first to volunteer.

It is hard for some medical personnel to stay

focused. Maybe it is because behind several years of schooling and years of treating patients, they find a stream of red tape, minor errors and lack of time which slightly clouds their way.

Red tape is usually caused whether directly or indirectly by the medical facility and/or insurance provider in efforts to cover themselves for a wide range of reasons. This, I believe, possibly influences some decisions made by medical professionals, which may cause them to take a different approach in doing their job or accomplishing their objectives. Often, at the expense of the patient's care.

I wish I did not have to be so critical of the medical community, but from 1975 to 1986 I worked in the medical field and today there seems to be a serious gap growing between recognizing or knowing the difference between an emergency and a non emergency, a serious situation and a not so serious situation, and good decisions versus bad decisions. I am confused about what has been going on in the medical community to cause such a change. Inept decisions are being made by professionals responsible for our well being, and we are forced to depend on them for help. Because they are experienced, we believe and depend on their decisions.

I am very much aware that over the years there have been hundreds, if not thousands, of malpractice lawsuits filed and won against the medical community. Also, we cannot remove the fact that there have been a lot of legitimate reasons for filing malpractice lawsuits and the patient who is too ill or too poor to file, just went away unnoticed. So in the end, guess who suffers? It's the next patient, that's who.

Along the way, there became the necessity to make

changes by insurance providers that seems to put caution and money first. An average bill for a month or two stay at an inpatient rehabilitation institute could run between thirty thousand and sixty thousand dollars or more and most people need a two month stay plus additional outpatient treatment. The outpatient rehab treatment works better for the patient who received the maximum inpatient therapy. If a patient is in inpatient therapy and is not responding well, it could very well be due to several reasons which include extent of the stroke, being under so much emotional stress that he/she cannot build any motivation, or the therapist not approaching the problem correctly in the first stages of therapy treatment. Either way the patient will be considered for a discharge before things become too expensive. The cost for home care or nursing home care for a year could be cheaper than one month of inpatient rehabilitation.

Take it from me because I know from experience, the difference between receiving enough inpatient and outpatient therapy and coming home and not receiving enough treatment before coming home. If not for my will and determination to get better, I would still be lying in bed unable to get up because when I came home after I had my third stroke March 23, 2009, I could not walk at all and barely had the strength to rise up in bed, but we'll get to that later in the book.

There are people who were possibly sent home from the hospital or emergency room too soon and either died or returned to the emergency department in worse shape. In the end the ones who benefited the most were the insurance providers and medical community more so than the patient because the insurance provider saved money, the medical personnel were paid on payday and the hospital submitted an invoice for payment of whatever services were given to whatever group that was paying. And the patient, if still alive, could quite possibly be dealing with the after affects of the decisions made that day, for the remainder of their life.

I have a lifelong friend whose family was severely affected by his son's stroke. His son died in 2003 at the age of twenty-four. He had no warning signs to suggest a stroke was imminent. He left behind two small sons and another on the way.

It was a February evening when he was taking a drive to Chicago. During the drive he developed a headache severe enough for him to pull off of the highway. He went to a hospital in Champagne Illinois.

During his emergency room visit, the normal procedures were followed for a person with a headache. After being unable to detect the real cause, he was sent on his way. Instead of continuing his drive, he decided to check into a hotel where he died overnight of an aneurysm.

This was a wakeup call to a lot of our family and friends because everyone felt the people affected by a stroke were generally further up in age.

I only hope that no one has to experience what I am dealing with, one year seven months, and fourteen days later, after the onset of my third stroke, when I was in the emergency room with no treatment whatsoever and admitted into a regular room and with absolutely no treatment for seven hours before the on call doctor arrived and gave me an aspirin and an MRI, but we'll get to that later in the book also.

The 'hurdles' facing a stroke survivor are high and

the necessity for seeking valuable help, information and knowledge are very important to maintain a better quality of life. That's where there's a need for people who can benefit from reading this book, or perhaps people who can share the knowledge of their recovery with other stroke survivors.

Well, I knew if I could write as much down as I could of my actual experiences, the highs and lows, and if people read it in full, they might see themselves in here. Then see that despite all of the dark days, there is a light at the end of the tunnel, and yes some tunnels are longer than others. So just stay true to yourself and stay motivated, put the work in, do not rush, and believe me you will get there, if not all the way, then close enough.

Chapter 2
A Showdown with Stroke #1
Only the Beginning

I have had three strokes, and each one was different. The first stroke was June 6, 2002, and brought on left side paralysis, speech impairment, vision confusion and memory loss.

I recall that morning very clearly. I had an appointment at one o'clock that afternoon. My intention was to get out of bed around eleven to begin preparation. I woke up at nine o'clock to go to the bathroom. I had a headache but decided not to take anything for it. I had been in the middle of a very good and serious dream so I wanted to get back to bed and hopefully resume it before it was time for me to get up. After falling back to sleep, I fell back into the same dream. There came a point where a gun was being pointed at me in the dream. It caused me to suddenly wake up. I noticed the clock had ten o'clock, and I still had a headache. My head ached so bad this time that I knew I had to take something for it right away.

I went to the bathroom, and for some reason which I cannot explain, I had to sit down this time. While sitting I felt something odd that affected my left arm. It was like I did not have a left arm. I immediately reached across to feel it, but it was not where I thought it was. I reached again and grabbed it, and I put it on my knee but something just was not right. To test myself, I looked away and reached for my left arm again and missed it slightly. I was confused by this because normally I would not have to look for the location of any body part before touching it.

I tried to think about it but it was very confusing so I just decided to go back to bed again. Then I felt something strange happening to my body. I reached for the house phone to call someone. I attempted to dial but I could not remember the first digit of a phone number to dial. I had a memory of at least ten different phone numbers in my head but at the onset of the stroke, which I did not know was a stroke at the time, I could not remember any portion of any telephone numbers. I grabbed my cellular phone and went to auto dial. Every number stored into the auto dialing section of my cellular phone looked like fours. By simply guessing I moved down to the fourth set of numbers and pushed the auto dial. Luckily my daughter, Tyan, answered. I told her about what was going on, and she said she was on her way. I realized the front door was locked. I had to basically drag myself to the door to unlock it because I was losing my ability to walk.

When she arrived from her house, which was just around the corner, we attempted to go to her car. At this time I was losing strength and became very heavy. She called my friend, Mike, who fortunately happened to be in the area at the time. He came right over. With Mike's help I made it to her car and she proceeded toward the hospital. After driving about seven blocks from the house, Tyan asked me which direction to go. I rose up to see where we were. I did see familiar surroundings, but I had no idea which way to go. I gave it some thought but I just could not remember. I have lived in this city all of my life but I could not remember what would have been very simple directions and only a ten minute drive or less.

Tyan took a guess on the directions herself and we made it to Centreville Hospital. After arriving at the emergency room I cannot remember a lot because events were a blur. I do remember having an MRI done which did not show anything. But all symptoms I displayed were that of someone having a stroke. At the time I did not ask any questions about anything because this was all new to me.

Next, I recall being in ICU and seeing the faces of my relatives. My father, who normally does not make hospital visits, was there every day. The next day I was able to acknowledge everything as though nothing had happened but I was aware that a stroke had occurred.

Each night in ICU the hospital staff would begin playing around like children on a playground. They would get so loud and out of hand that I could not get any sleep. The first few nights I did not complain because I believed things would change. Finally one night I had to call for the person in charge. I asked if this was really the intensive care unit of the hospital and she said *yes*. I recognized her voice as being one of the people that I heard clowning around, so I did not call her again. After several nights of this I asked my sister, Lillie, if she would get me transferred to St. Louis University Hospital.

After spending a week at Centreville Hospital, where in my right mind I would never have gone for any reason, not to mention that St. Mary's Hospital was less than five minutes from my home, I was finally transferred.

The following day while waiting for my transfer, the only hospital personnel to show up in my room was the person who brought breakfast and lunch. It seemed as though they were disappointed about my decision to transfer and could not show their faces. I did not know if they were embarrassed or pissed off. The only thing I really was sure about was that I did not want to spend another night at Centreville Hospital.

After arriving at St. Louis University Hospital, I was given a CT SCAN and an MRI and was diagnosed as having an aneurysm which did not require surgery.

I spent another week at St. Louis University Hospital. Before I could be assigned into a rehabilitation program, all affects of the stroke had disappeared and I was back to normal without therapy. Actually, I do not know when I was able to walk again because for the two weeks spent between hospitals I did hardly any walking. I do recall my speech was back to normal immediately and my arms worked fine a day or so after the stroke. I did not have a speech, vision or memory problem anymore. I was released from St. Louis University Hospital with no symptoms whatsoever of a stroke.

I considered myself to be very lucky, even though I did not understand what was going on at the time. I had no idea this first stroke was a warning. Even though thirty years earlier I had heard that strokes come in six month intervals, I still had nothing to base it on so there was no worrying on my part.

I returned to my job as Demolition Coordinator for St. Clair County and resumed other activities like playing basketball and volleyball. Thinking back about everything that happened, I should have changed a lot of things in my life. I never had a personal doctor to consult for advice because in the past I had never needed one. I was never sick enough for a doctor's visit, so I never got concerned enough about what happened. The longest I kept a common cold was three days, and if I caught the flu I would nurse it for a week or so and I cleared up just fine.

Since I was given a clean bill of health from the hospital and some diet information, I thought my life was back to normal. I was never advised on what the possibilities were for another stroke. I did not know the things to do and what not to do. As a matter of fact, I was in slight denial that I had a stroke. I really did not know what had happened, because I thought an actual stroke would have been more severe. I have only recently learned about the type of stroke I had.

I was given a list of dietary foods to implement into my eating routine, but I knew nothing and learned nothing about strokes. I guess by getting off so easy and being healthy all of my life I was not able to give more respect to the warning I had been given. I should have acquired a doctor, changed my diet, monitored my blood pressure, had my cholesterol checked, and the list could go on and on.

Years of studying and a hundred questions later, I have learned many causes of strokes. I have learned that a stroke is an illness to part of the brain. When a stroke happens, the blood that feeds part of the brain is cut off. This means damage can happen to the brain tissue in that area. When brain cells die during a stroke, abilities controlled by that area of the brain are lost. These abilities may include speech, movement, and memory. The way a stroke affects you depends on where the stroke occurs in the brain and how much of the brain is damaged.

I did not know that after my second stroke I would dedicate my life to studying strokes and their affects to the brain and to the body.

It was not until after my second stroke that I became concerned enough to seek out every bit of information I could about strokes. After years of studying at libraries and questioning doctors and medical professionals, I now know that the first stroke I had was a mini-stroke. A mini-stroke happens when the brain's blood supply is temporarily interrupted. The symptoms are similar to a full stroke except the symptoms are temporary and disappear within 24 hours. Even though the symptoms may disappear, the risks of having a more serious stroke in the future are highly increased.

Cleothus Bell

Chapter 3
Should've, Would've, Could've
My Regrets

Sometimes during a healthy or young person's lifetime little if any thought is given to the possibility of a severe illness affecting them. There exists this notion of being exempt from disabling injuries, diseases and illnesses. Being young and healthy, our immediate concerns are often the way we feel at the present time. We seem to leave tomorrow's feelings to be handled tomorrow.

Growing up I was always active in sports. I loved to play tennis, basketball and volleyball, but my eating habits were terrible. I had a love for almost any food on the market. It did not matter whether it was home cooking, fast food or major restaurants; I never drew a line on where to go or what to eat and what time of day to eat it. Even though I knew about arterial sclerosis, high blood pressure, diabetes and numerous other conditions that can alter a person's future, like a considerable amount of others, I did not think it could ever happen to me. I always heard about the things that were not good for the body like eating a lot of red meat, high calorie, high sodium, and high in fat foods. Each time I heard someone speaking about these things I would listen but I thought it was a crock of bull. I did not realize that living a better life today could help assure good health tomorrow.

One of my sayings about life was to *live life so as to not have regrets once you get old*. Sometimes regrets can be something as small as not taking that vacation you always wanted, or not getting away for a while when you were able to. Other regrets come from the fact that you did not do the right thing before something went wrong.

My biggest regret, "Should've, would've, could've," came after my first stroke.

I *should've* acquired a doctor, which *would've* been the beginning of regular blood pressure screening, monitoring my cholesterol levels and changing my diet, which *could've* prevented the second stroke that changed my life and my family's life forever.

While being physically active is good for one's mental and physical health, it is equally as important to do what is necessary to maintain a healthy diet, reduce high blood pressure, lower your cholesterol levels, and manage stress. This could cut your risk of heart disease and stroke considerably.

There is a tremendous lack of knowledge about strokes which creates a misunderstanding, which may lead people to underestimate the severity of a stroke and the affect it can have on you and your family. Many people do not realize there is a great deal that can be done to change the future for people affected by strokes.

There is a huge amount of information that exists today to show how we can prevent tens of thousands of strokes each year, save thousands from dying because of a stroke, reduce the number of people with severe disability due to stroke, and increase the success rate for independence of stroke survivors.

There is a growing need for more medical staff in emergency and non-emergency areas of hospitals to have a better awareness in identifying and responding to the early detection of a stroke victim.

Chapter 4
A Showdown with Stroke #2
Nothing Will Ever Be the Same

My second stroke happened six months after my first stroke on December 2, 2002. It caused left side paralysis, speech impairment and a blood pressure reading of 220/180.

That particular morning I actually had gotten out of bed and was just standing around like I would do on a normal morning. I slightly leaned on the bed and stood there for a minute. I felt nothing odd or abnormal. It started out like any other morning. I sat on the side of the bed and I still felt fine. When I stood back up and attempted to take a step, I began to fall. I immediately started hopping on one leg to prevent the fall. I fell against a large vase and then into the wall. I attempted to push myself from the wall but was unsuccessful because my left arm, which was against the wall, would not move. I called out to my girlfriend, Kim, who was home from work at this time. She came into the room, grabbed my right hand and pulled me from against the wall. She then proceeded to help me to the bed while I hopped on one foot. I told her to call an ambulance because I thought I was having a stroke.

I attempted to put on a sweater while sitting on the bed, but I fell to the floor. While I was on the floor, I began to realize that I had not done the right things for myself after having the mini-stroke. I began hitting the floor in disgust. At this time I did not feel bad physically or mentally. I only felt weakness in my left arm and leg.

This time I was taken by ambulance to Barnes

Jewish Hospital in St. Louis. While in the emergency room, I recall being surrounded by lots of hospital personnel. Everyone looked busy and intense. At one time I recall vaguely shaking uncontrollably. I thought it was from the chill in the air but I was told later that I had a seizure, and I was administered medication for it.

An MRI and a CT SCAN were done. The tests came back, and I was diagnosed with having had a hemorrhagic stroke. The doctor explained that the hemorrhagic stroke was caused by an aneurysm which had some leakage of blood but did not require surgery. Hemorrhagic strokes are less common but more deadly than ischemic strokes.

After hearing this, a lot of memories from the past surfaced. I knew about this type of stroke because in 1969, at the age of twenty my girlfriend died after having had what was called a brain hemorrhage. Back then I had never heard the word stroke and the diagnosis of a brain hemorrhage were like hearing words from the Greek vocabulary.

I do not recall the actual amount of time I spent in the emergency room. Frankly, I do not remember too much of anything about that entire day. I do recall briefly waking up and seeing the faces of my family. The next thing I remember was that night had fallen, and I was taken to the room where I would spend the next two months at the Rehabilitation Institute. Before being put in bed I was weighed. My normal weight was 223 pounds, but now the scale showed my weight as 185 pounds. You can imagine the thoughts that raced through my mind as I thought of how, in a matter of hours, I had lost thirty-eight pounds.

This all happened on a Friday and therapy

treatment was scheduled to begin on Monday morning. I spent the following days trying to assess the damage that had been inflicted on me by the stroke and trying to figure out why I felt so bad. I could not feel or move anything on my left side. I had this enormous amount of pressure all over my body. What I was feeling was so unpleasant and intolerable that my thoughts were that I would not wish this feeling even on my worse enemy.

That same weekend there was a fire drill, and everyone in every room had to come out into the hallway for a while. I have to say, this was a blessing for my thoughts because like the saying goes, regardless of how bad you are doing, there is always someone doing worse. I got the opportunity to see that during the time I spent in that hallway. Afterward, I was able to get control of my thoughts about my situation a little bit better.

The first few days at the Rehabilitation Institute, I merely went through the routine I was put through by the therapists. I was so weak from the stroke that I really was not able to assist or help in my therapy in any way. My mind was lacking in clarity and organization. I could not clearly express my thoughts and as a result of the stroke I had difficulty understanding the things that were happening around me. I felt like I was enclosed inside a box. I was unable to express my thoughts or feelings, so everything I could see was accepted the way it was.

For five days per week at an average of four hours per day I received physical therapy two hours, occupational therapy for one hour, speech for thirty minutes and neurological therapy for thirty minutes, including plenty of exercise.

Because of the quick and simple recovery I had from the previous stroke, I was also dealing with the belief of an immediate and easy recovery. I was thinking my body would heal like it did with the previous stroke. I had no idea what was lurking around the corner for me.

It seemed as though I was looking at everything from a rear seat. I was fortunate the therapists were doing a great job because mentally and physically I was in bad shape. I could see the therapists consulting each other, teaming up and changing up. I was amazed at their team effort. I remember the times when two people assisted me while I tried to walk. One guy was drenched in sweat before we were done. He looked so worn out and I felt sorry for him, but there was absolutely nothing I could do to help.

My body had the most unbearable and miserable feeling. A feeling that was agonizing, but since there was no pain it seemed useless of me to complain. I guess the stroke caused all or most of the muscles in my body to collapse, which caused me to feel pressure from my ribcage. The lack of trunk muscles made it feel like I was carrying around dead weight. Sitting in a wheel chair was quite uncomfortable because I felt like I had a hundred pounds of weight sitting in my lap. The weight of my body in the chair caused me to feel every rod running through the chair. The only time I felt at ease was when lying flat on my back in bed.

My left arm and leg had no life at all. One day I attempted to move in the wheelchair but it would not move. I tried a little harder but I felt a sharp pain in my left shoulder. I reached to grab my shoulder and saw that my arm had fallen from the arm board attached to the chair. The reason the chair would not move was because my hand had become lodged in the sports of the wheel. I understood now, though a little too late, the importance of using the Velcro strap that was hooked to the arm board. My arm sometimes would fall off to the side and being lifeless and with absolutely no feeling could have become severely damaged without me being aware of it.

Chapter 5
A Friend Within
Depression versus Determination

After working continuously everyday and not seeing or feeling much improvement, I finally grasped that the quick healing process that occurred after my first stroke had been truly a blessing, but this time around I was not going to be that lucky. I also had hope because there was another patient in therapy that had a stroke and both of his legs were affected, yet after two weeks; he was walking around and kidding like nothing had ever happened. Seeing and knowing this also helped to fuel my thoughts of a miracle recovery.

When the truth of my situation began to weigh in on me, I felt like the real world had opened up a merciless door on me. My thoughts and hopes of a miraculous recovery were shattered.

I tell you, the state of mind I was in at the time was no joking matter. I was devastated to realize the situation I was in, and knowing that I could not do anything about it only made it that much worse. I began feeling as though I was sinking into a dark hole, and if you were not in the hole with me then you could not help. I felt the people around could not relate to me because no matter how skilled and how much training they had, they had not experienced what I was going through and the feelings I was having, so how could they be capable of helping me.

As time passed, I lost my desire to do anything. If what I did in therapy did not show instant progress, I felt that it was useless to continue. Soon, I became extremely depressed. I could not fight it off because I was not aware that it needed to be fought off. I could barely find the energy to get out of bed. The only time my mind was at peace was when I had a visit from a friend or a family member. During their visits I never talked about how I felt, and I really do not know why. I did complain a lot about some of the things that went on in therapy, as if I was an expert on what the therapist should be doing.

During the day I began to make up stupid excuses to avoid therapy. I used excuses like, *I've got company coming, and I need to see them.* The depression became so bad I actually thought about things I never dreamed I could think about or imagine. My life became so senseless and useless that the thought of taking my own life was a simple remedy. That kind of thinking was hard for me to believe, but it proves that my mind was a wreck. All I wanted to do was to go home. I did not want therapy anymore. In my mind everything was going wrong. I wanted to go home just to see if the thoughts of suicide would still exist.

Fearing the unknown is one of the worse feelings I think a person can go through in their life, and that is exactly what I was going through at the time. I could not see a way out of the darkness.

When I received a visitor I continued to complain about the goings on at the institute and about whatever I did not understand. I needed help but I did not have a clue where to begin or who to go to for answers. I had never in my wildest dreams contemplated taking my own life, and so there was no way I could mention it to anyone. It was my deep, dark, secret.

Things changed one morning while I prepared to wash my face. I caught a glimpse of myself in the mirror.

The person I saw, I did not like. I stared at myself. The first thing I noticed was my matted and tangled hair. My eyes drooped down like a sad face. My skin looked dark and crusty. I looked like I had aged forty years. I was a fifty-two year old man but I looked ninety-two. I simply looked a wreck. This was the strangest thing to see.

All my life I kept myself well groomed from head to toe. I had performed a plenty of fashion shows where I was the one receiving the loudest cheers and garnered a lot of loyal followers. I had been offered modeling jobs in the past but I passed on them. There were not too many days in my life when I looked like a bum except for yard work days. I had never let myself go like this. I knew I was sick but I still could not imagine ever looking like the man staring back at me in the mirror.

After seeing myself this way and trying to come to grips with what I saw, I had to realize it was me and I was in bad shape. I began to feel sad then sorry for the person I saw in the mirror. I did not know the next move to make so I continued to stare. It became the saddest thing to see, and it was me. The man in the mirror reminded me of a homeless person that had lived on the street for a lifetime with no desire to do any better.

I saw myself as a man facing disappointment; a man who had thrown in the towel on life. For me, this was unfamiliar territory and for the first time in my life I did not have an answer. I was at a point in life that I had never reached. I had no questions, and I had no answers. I was afraid of myself. I could not share my thoughts with anyone. The one thing I did was to make another appointment with the mirror and soon.

Later, when I crept back to the mirror I sat there

quietly. I did not know what to say or think. I just stared at myself. Believe it or not, I was afraid, terrified and speechless. The staring grew deeper and I had to force myself to stay. I began thinking, and my thinking got deeper.

I do not know how much time passed but finally the fear of the man in the mirror began to fade. I finally grew calm. I sat and observed and rationalized my situation. I started to feel a breakthrough coming. I slowly separated myself from the man I was looking at in the mirror, and I started seeing the person in the mirror as a separate human being, someone that was in need of my help, and someone that needed guidance. I said *your body is a wreck, man.* And then things started to come together.

I began to realize it was my body that was in bad shape, not my mind. The door was beginning to open. For a lifetime this body has been in perfect health. It has been able to do everything I asked of it. It has taken me any and everywhere I have wanted to go without any physical problems, and now it needs my help. Now is the time for me to give back. I stared even closer in the mirror, almost eyes touching eyes. A voice rang out and said loudly, "M.....f....r it's time for you to get up off your ass and get to work. Nobody can do this but you. You have a responsibility to yourself, now do it. The lights were suddenly turned on. From that day forward I refused to complain about anything.

Every morning at six o'clock, I got up, raised the bed and waited on my breakfast. Regardless of how it tasted, I ate every bit of it. I told myself that my body needs this first meal to have enough nourishment to get through my therapy.

Soon, I found the ability to do things without the need for as much help as before. I became determined to get all of my hygiene done in the morning with as little assistance as possible. In just a few days and with absolutely no assistance at all, I got it done. In no time I was getting into the wheelchair and wheeling to the therapy room on my own, because I could not wait on the therapist anymore. My right arm and leg worked fine and that was enough for me to roll out. The therapist would meet me sometimes in the hall wheeling in the chair and would just smile with approval. Pretty soon I was arriving in the therapy room too early because I wanted to begin therapy as soon as possible. I had only one thing to say when I reached the therapy room – "Who's working with me today?"

Therapists finally stopped coming to my room to get me. They knew that I would be to therapy on my own. The more I worked the better I felt. At the end of some days I would be dog tired, but I felt great on the inside. Some days when I had completed my therapy and there was still time on the clock, the therapist would ask me if there was anything special I wanted to do? My response would always be, "Yes. I would like to walk the stairs." Walking the stairs was difficult, but I welcomed the challenge.

I learned how to conquer my fears and my depression. I have learned that many people who survive a stroke feel the same way: fear, frustration, anger, sadness and a sense of pity over their physical and mental losses. These feelings are a natural response to the effects of a stroke. Depression is a sense of hopelessness that disrupts a person's ability to function. It is common among most individuals after a stroke.

Depression can be treated and the faster you are treated, the better. It is important to recognize the signs and get help fast.

Today I know that it is normal to feel tired and discouraged at times after having had a stroke. But it is more important to notice your progress and take pride in each step you make. Feeling sad about having a stroke and the resulting disabilities are normal. But if you let depression take complete control of your thoughts, it can interfere with your recovery. I want you to know and realize that it does not matter how far along you may have come in your recovery, depression, if not addressed in time, can bring a halt to whatever progress is needed to assure a better future for you.

At the first signs of depression, talk to yourself, with your family or your doctor about what you are feeling. There may even be another stroke survivor hanging in the wings with a good attitude and willing to talk to you. Early treatment for depression can help prevent a delay in recovery.

Some warning signs of depression are feelings of sadness, guilt, worthlessness or hopelessness. Also the loss of interest in activities you used to enjoy, fatigue or loss of energy, and possibly the most critical sign, thoughts of suicide or death.

At night in bed, whenever I went over the day's events in my mind, I sometimes reached a point of thinking where I would get stuck on a particular thought, and without any advanced warning I would feel depression settling in. As time passed, I began to get a handle on Mr. Depression. And as soon as I realized I was beginning to think of mood swinging thoughts, I offset them with pleasant ones. Sometimes I would find a comedy show on TV. For the first time ever, I ran across the Jerry Seinfeld Show one night. It happened to come on at ten o'clock every night, about the same time depressing thoughts would often set in. I started watching it and it really helped me. After my stay in rehabilitation and even now, I still watch the show almost every night.

As time passed, I grew more accustomed to the voice of motivation inside my head. It grew into a lasting friendship within, which still exists today. I began feeling like I had a friend inside or *a friend within*.

At times, it became funny because my therapist did not know where my new found energy level generated from. Once, while attempting to do a strenuous workout, the therapist observed me encouraging myself. She looked at me with seriousness all over her face and asked me if I was okay. I told her, that I was fine and I was telling myself that I could do it. She said, 'That's good, keep it up.'

The therapists worked hard and showed their appreciation of my desire to work hard. They applied themselves as though their lives depended on my recovery. Due to my hard work and the determination of all the therapists I made a great deal of improvement.

You must know and follow your rehabilitation plan. Most people find that rehabilitation is hard work but a slow process. Tasks and activities that were once easy for you before often become more difficult after a stroke, but know that this is the beginning of your new life and these first steps can be the most important of your new journey.

After a month of inpatient rehabilitation I was granted four more weeks of therapy. The upcoming four weeks were to become the most challenging of my life. There were tons of routines to work on, and at times they did not seem to have any reference to my getting better. Even though the process was working I could not help wishing for it to come faster.

I was reassigned to a therapist I had worked with in the early weeks of my rehabilitation. His squat routines had me sweating and exhausted. The first two days I wanted to complain because I felt like he was picking on me. I felt that since he knew I was a hard worker that he wanted to challenge me to get totally exhausted. Little did he know, but after a pep talk from *my friend within* I began looking forward to working with him. Soon I did not want to stop unless sweat was falling from my chin. Pretty soon I found myself lifting from the chair and from the bed a lot easier than before.

I was also assigned another physical therapist that had me doing a great deal of walking with a wide-bottom quad cane. Before I started walking, while lying on my back she would stretch my hamstrings until she was exhausted. After a few days of this, she was able to push my leg towards my head until it almost touched my face. She would ask me if I was okay and my response would be "that feels good."

The stairs became my favorite place to walk. As we progressed and I became stronger, I asked her to separate her position from me more, which gave me a more independent feeling. As days passed the separation grew farther and farther, until she was confident enough to wait at the bottom of each flight of stairs. These were proud days for me and for her.

My walking was better with someone holding the belt, but I never walked solo without holding on to something, until one Saturday, on a therapy off day. I went to the gym alone. One of the technicians happened to be there straightening up around the place. I asked her if she would monitor me while I stood and picked up some weights from the floor. She agreed and placed the weights for me. Each time I picked them up, I would take about two steps to the next set. She told me to widen my feet more when taking a step. Well that Saturday was one of the most exciting days of my journey, because when I widened my stand I was able to walk without anymore assistance and with almost total balance.

I have to say, that was one of the most changing days of my journey to recovery. And to think, that Saturday was actually an off day. No therapists were working and no one was in the gym other than me and the technician. A technician's job was to keep things sanitary in the gym and they sometimes would assist therapists in working with patients. This changing day was made possible because *my friend within* encouraged me to go to the gym on an off day.

After completing an additional four weeks of inpatient therapy, on January 27, 2003 I was released from inpatient rehabilitation to go home. I was granted outpatient therapy downstairs in the same facility. By this time, I was walking with a single leg cane, climbing five flights of stairs without getting tired, standing and cooking in the center's kitchen.

During days of group sessions, we often had the opportunity to stand before the class and share whatever we wanted. During one class in particular I spoke about a program I had seen a few days before on TV. It was a program about racing with large tractors. There was a man in the race who had both legs amputated above the knee. He inspired me because my thoughts went back to the feelings he must have had after his surgery and what it took for him to weather the storm and get to the point of being on a one hundred thousand dollar piece of equipment in a race. I thought surely if he had this type of money, he could easily have just laid around every day and take life easy. I told the class that the courage and determination the man showed was very motivating to me.

After classes, sometimes the therapists would have a private meeting with me to tell me how much they appreciated what I was saying because there were other patients in the session that needed to hear the things I talked about.

After I spoke about the amputee, a therapist told me that we had a very depressed amputee who was sitting in the class. Therapists had been attempting to get through to her. They were happy with the speech I presented because they said it touched the lady amputee like nothing else could have.

I was also asked where I had learned to speak so well before a crowd because I took total command of the microphone and the podium. My response was that I only spoke what I felt.

Soon after, I was recommended to participate in a physical therapy treatment session with a class of future therapists at Washington University. Afterwards, I was supposed to speak to the class. I was also paid for my time and services which made things even better! In the class there were at least one hundred fifty students. I must admit I was sort of nervous but when I saw I had everyone's attention, the nervousness went away.

After my second stroke, I received a great deal of cognitive exercises to insure there were no neurological affects from the stroke. For two hours each day I received mind blowing work sheets with problem solving exercises. The worksheet exercises were extremely hard but I was determined to solve every one I was given. At times I felt drained, because I became so engrossed into whatever the formula was and upon completing them I always received a grade of one-hundred. Each day the therapist challenged me with worksheets that seemed to be harder than the previous one. One day at the rehab institute my daughter came early to pick me up and I showed her what I was working on. After reading it, she immediately handed it back and said, "I have no idea what this is about." I said, "this is what I get graded on every day." I told her about the day I was confused about what was on a work sheet and gave it back. The therapist read it and could not figure it out either. I got the worksheet back from the therapist and I figured it out. This was the day she began to respect the good scores I had been receiving. She always had the answer sheet to grade the worksheets, so there was not a reason for her to search through the formula for the answer.

One day a therapist gave me a worksheet with squares on it. In about a hundred of the squares were X marks. On a clean sheet of squares she wanted me to put an X mark in each box, identical to the other sheet. Once I started, it seemed like an impossible task to line them up in the identical locations. Once I started, I began to develop a pattern and in no time I was finished. For the entire time she was sitting in front of me. When I handed her the paper she asked if I had checked my work. I told her that I did not need to because everything was correct. I was not trying to be cocky, I just felt as though I had every box checked correctly. Her facial expression was one of doubt, but once she checked my sheet against her sheet, she told me every check was in the correct square. She said no one had ever gotten every box correct and no one had ever finished in eleven minutes. She said I should still check my work.

On another occasion, Kim and I were at the laundromat, and I was going through my yearly routine of putting a schedule together for a dart league I had been running. The league consisted of twenty teams, and the season lasted for twenty weeks before the playoffs began. Each season, teams were divided into two conferences and four divisions. Each section had to be matched to represent divisional games, conference games and also road and home games at an equal basis for each team. Each season there were mistakes in the scheduling, and a new schedule had to be made after the corrections were made. Sometimes the last few weeks of the schedule were not released until the season was almost over.

While sitting in the laundromat, I decided to start working on the schedule. At home I would type everything into the computer and begin putting things in order. At this time I only had a pencil and paper. Once I started writing team names down, I started matching teams and a pattern seemed to develop. When I started working on it, I could not stop. When I finished, only two hours had passed and I had written a twenty week schedule. After checking it I did not find any errors. Each team was matched perfectly. I went home and after transferring it to the computer and furnishing a complete twenty week schedule to every team in the dart league, there were no complaints of mistakes for the entire season. For the first time in twelve seasons I did not receive one complaint about the schedule. I was relieved and pleased.

Lots of other things began to happen this way, but it was not something I could share with too many people. This is not something people will understand or believe. I did not understand it myself until I was looking at a special program on television late one night. The program was about strokes and the affects it can have on the brain. It talked about the different areas of the brain and its development after losing the usage of one side. They added that when the left side of the brain begins to shut off, the right side begins to function. It was said that we use only half of the brain anyway, which is the left side. The right side of the brain increases in development when something causes the left side to fail. The right side of the brain is the smarter half of the brain.

After watching the program, I thought back to the days in the rehabilitation program, when I went through the neurological programs and exercise formulas. I wondered if working with the different cognitive skills techniques was what triggered the development process. I had the choice to tell my therapist at each session that the formulas were too hard and they would have let it go at that. Each day at the institute, I saw and felt how difficult the formula solving exercises were, but I viewed it as another challenge.

Chapter 6
Nine Months of Botox With No Results
Painful But True

At the end of my first month of outpatient therapy, I was approved for a second month. Every step was still a challenge, but I met each one with no complaints. However, I still had problems with the muscles tightening in my left arm. These muscles, located on the interior fold of the arm, caused my arm to pull upwards. During therapy sessions, it was extremely difficult whenever I attempted exercises that required arm extension. Also my hamstrings dominated my quad muscles in my leg, preventing me from making a full extension of my left leg.

The therapist prescribed a muscle relaxer but I did not like the side effects and the feeling of being 'high' on medication, so I stopped taking the medication. I was then recommended for Botox injections, which would target the specific muscles that were dominating. The Botox injections were arranged, but not until my third month of outpatient rehabilitation. The doctor was in the same facility but I could only receive the injections every three months. The first set of injections consisted of about twelve shots in my arm and about nine shots into my hamstrings. It goes without saying that this was not a pleasant day for me. My thoughts were that I was ready to do anything to get more mobility from my leg and more movement from my arm. The pain I had to go through was a simple step in order to achieve more independence.

I was told by the doctor in April 2003 that the

medication would take about seven days to take effect, but as of September 2010, over seven years later I still have not experienced the relaxing affect of the Botox. The therapist in occupational therapy was supposed to talk to the doctor about it not working because she needed it done to continue my occupational therapy. But, by this time I was in my final month of outpatient therapy, and there was no time or a reason to inquire.

By the time I was ready for the second round of Botox injections I was at home, however I still wanted to resume taking the injections. This was July of 2003, and since I am on the subject of the second Botox visit I must add some of the events that happened during the visit.

When I arrived for my appointment I was sent to a treatment room. During this visit a guy looking to be in his early twenties came in and began examining my leg and arm as though he was putting together an evaluation for treatment. Even though I had not seen him before, nor had this type of procedure been done on me before, I did not have a reason to question the procedures. A short time later, my doctor came in. As she was filling the containers for the injections, the assistant began discussing a few things with the doctor about the examination of my arm and leg. The room was the normal size of a small examination room in a doctor's office so I heard every word. While the doctor placed the amount of medicine in her bottles like before, the assistant asked about the dosages being placed in the bottles because some of the dosages were not as high as the others. The doctor explained to the assistant that she had one more patient to see and she wanted to be sure there was enough to go around. After hearing her response, I wondered about her intentions, because her explanation did not sound right. Especially since my previous Botox session was ineffective. Believe me when I say that I got absolutely no response from the previous treatments. And because the medication did not take effect, my last month of outpatient occupational therapy did not go as well as planned. The therapist was surprised by the lack of results also, but nothing could be done at that time because the outpatient treatment time had expired.

In another conversation she asked the young assistant how he was coming along with his invoices. He went on to tell her how they looked so far on his computer. After listening a while I began wondering if he was a relative of hers. I began looking closer at the guy. His dress was wrinkled trousers and worn-out sneakers. To me he appeared to be a student. I was not sure but my gut feelings were that something was not right. Believe it or not this Botox session did not work either.

After a few months, I received a statement in the mail of the first two sessions which had been paid by the insurance company. The statement showed a charge of $3,300 for the first treatment and $4,400 for the second session.

After three months, I returned for a third Botox treatment. I let the doctor know again the treatments had not worked, and again there was no clarification given. This time my daughter, Tyan, was in the room with me. Again nothing happened as far as muscle relaxation. I am by no means a specialist on the treatment of the Botox drug, but there is one thing I am sure of, and that is, if this drug was injected by a specialist directly into the muscle area to relax the muscle, then it should have had some type of affect on that muscle or someone should have been able to explain to me why it did not. At this point I had to wonder about what was really going on. A doctor at a rehabilitation institute administers Botox injections several times to a patient but it does not work on the patient. I had to wonder what was really going on. Was I the only one this happened to?

The injections were very painful but I do not know why they did not work. From the beginning, the doctor said the first session was sort of an experimental session to determine what amount was needed to do the job. All I can say is that her experimentation never got right for the treatment, but it sure was right on the money when the invoices of $3,300, $4,400 and $3,300 were submitted to the insurance provider for payment. There were three visits in a nine month period. I finally decided I'd had enough, and I never returned.

Just for the record, I should have done more as far as voicing my disapproval of these events and taking things to a higher level. But I had been through a lot in the past twelve months and my complaining days were behind me. My days ahead had been shifted into complete recovery mode. I could not dwell on the past because I was concentrating on my future.

Chapter 7
Back Home after Stroke #2
Back to Work and Working Out

After completing outpatient therapy I was able to manage most things on my own at home. By this time my walking was okay, except for long distances. I knew this was just the beginning of my journey. Compared to what I had been through, I felt humble, grateful, proud and lucky to be where I was.

When you return home after a stroke, you will need to make sure you are able to take care of yourself or have someone who is willing to help care for you. Your daily living has to be under control. An important part of that is daily self-care, which will include choosing the right type of clothes. In doing so you should choose your clothes to make getting dressed easier. Also what you choose to wear should reflect who you are and how you are feeling.

To get dressed, use your unaffected arm to dress the affected side first. To undress, take the clothing off the unaffected side first and then remove it from the affected side.

Use a long handled shoehorn to put on shoes. You may also want to use a device to help put on your socks. Visit a local medical supply store and browse around. Talk to the store attendant for helpful advice.

When you are choosing clothes, try avoiding tight fitting sleeves, arm holes, pant legs and waistlines. Look for clothes that fasten in front. They are often easier to manage. Replace buttons, zippers, and shoelaces with velcro fasteners. Choose coats and jackets lined with slippery fabrics like satin, silk or nylon. They are easier to put on than unlined garments. Look for fabrics that wrinkle less, so you will not have to iron as much.

You may have experienced changes in the way you walk after a stroke. These changes can eventually lead to problems with your feet. You can avoid most of these problems by checking your feet every day for cracks, blisters, sores, swelling or any changes in skin color. This is especially important if you have diabetes, circulation problems or reduced feeling in your feet. Any sign of infection, such as redness, swelling, or discharge, should be examined by your family doctor right away.

Always wear socks. Socks made of wool help absorb perspiration and keep the feet cool and dry. Buy shoes that are wide and deep enough, and fit snugly at the heel. Ideal shoes for stroke patients have low heels, and shock absorbing soles, Velcro fasteners, deep, rounded toe boxes, and leather or canvas uppers. When shopping for shoes, do so at the end of the day when your feet are naturally swollen. Be sure to have both feet measured. Keep toe nails trimmed.

Support your affected arm on a lap tray or on a device called an arm trough when you are sitting. If you can, use your other hand to position the affected hand. It should be in front of you, with the fingers opened and the wrist supported. Use foam wedges or arm supports placed on the tray to raise the hand. This reduces swelling. Gently bend and open the fingers of your affected hand with your other hand. Gently stroke the back of the hand and wrist if your hand is tightly closed or spastic. Do not force it open. This should help the fingers to relax.

Before your stroke, you may have had a preference

for using a shower or bathtub. After your stroke, you may find that you have to adapt to a routine that is safe and allows you as much independence as possible. You should look into installing grab bars near the tub and shower. Put non-skid tape or a suction mat on the bottom of bathtubs and showers. If you find it hard to safely get in and out of the bathtub, think about a tub bench and a handheld, flexible shower hose.

Get everything ready that you will need before your bath. Collect towels, clothing, soaps, and shampoos before you get wet. Test the water before getting in. If you have decreased feeling on one side of the body, you might not notice that the water may be too hot.

Try using soap on a rope, a bath mitt and a long handled brush. Decide on a sponge bath if getting in and out of the bathtub or shower is unsafe.

It is common to feel shoulder pain on the side affected by the stroke. This happens when one arm is weak and hangs down without any support. It can lead to a shoulder problem called frozen shoulder. This is why it is important to keep your arm supported when you are standing or sitting.

Make sure you are eating enough to fuel your body. Drink plenty of fluids. Plan your day to take advantage of the times when you have the most energy.

Every day, make a list of the things you want to do and try to see them through. Decide which jobs are the most important to you. On days when you feel tired, do only the things you must. On high energy days, you can work your way a little further down the list. Take short rest breaks when you become tired. If you nap during the day, keep your naps short. Save your longest sleep for the night. Try to go to sleep and wake up at the same time.

At home I began walking inside everyday and pretty soon to the corner every day. After a few weeks I could walk half the entire block and then the whole block. Eventually the time came when I could walk a square block radius that included a total of eight blocks.

In the coming months and years I still had the limp in my left leg and limited use of my left arm but I had no complaints. My sporting activities were no more but I was able to go back to work as the County Demolition Coordinator.

Not long after starting back to work, I lost my private insurance coverage. I applied for and was granted Medicaid and S.S.I. Months later the coverage from Medicare became available.

Because of the fear of having another stroke, I had to give up my career job because I felt the need to have insurance was greater. Even though I did not think the quality of service in the medical world would be the same as having private insurance, my main concern at this time was to have some type of insurance just in case I had another stroke. I figured something was better than nothing.

The one thing I learned the hard way about insurance was that the medical community seemed to give more and faster service to a person with private insurance. I also learned that with government insurance you had better be prepared for some of the shabby care from institutions that are supposed to be there for your care. What can you expect when something is free? Knowing what I know now, I think I would have been better off trying to find another private insurer. I guess I was kind of living in the fear of going through another stroke and not having insurance. I also knew that having a stroke had added a negative notch to my medical history. There was a fear of being on the pre-existing list and being denied insurance coverage.

After making a request, my new doctor scheduled me for additional therapy in the outpatient rehabilitation facility at Memorial Hospital. After completing one month of physical therapy I was told that I would be released from there because there may be a problem receiving a payment from the insurance provider. The occupational therapy continued for another month and before it ended I was setting the table with my left hand, which was a lot better than before.

Note: If you are a stroke patient, I cannot stress enough the importance of attending every minute of therapy, whether it is in a rehabilitation program or while you are in your home. Learn what you are to do from the therapist, because their time with you is temporary, and your insurance provider has a limited amount of money it will pay towards your recovery.

Even though the odds may seem to be against you, even when others are in doubt about your future, and sometimes when you are in doubt yourself, remember that *determination*, *motivation* and *perseverance* can turn the table of hope in your favor.

With the money I had saved I joined a gym and paid $500 upfront for the membership in full. Not because I could afford it, rather because I did not know how my financial situation would be in the coming months, and I did not want any interruptions during my workouts. I paid the full price also because I wanted the option to go any day of the week and any time of the day with no restrictions. I wanted the complete freedom of exercising whenever I wanted and to stop when I got ready.

I would schedule a workout at the gym everyday and if I was exhausted after twenty or thirty minutes I would quit and go home. I knew if I tried to do too much, it would discourage me from going on a regular basis. I eventually began to feel better movement in my limbs even though it was tiring work.

It felt really good and relaxing to be there because I was able to go at the times when there weren't a lot of people around using the equipment and I could then try everything out. Plus I had kind of a self-conscious feeling about my disability when there was a large group of people occupying the gym. For some reason I felt as though I was in the way because everyone was physically fit and also I felt people were watching me because of my working out with my disability.

After a few weeks I was able to open the big door leading to the outside with my left hand. I say this because this was a large hydraulic door and I had to grab and push the lever while opening the door to exit the building. The coordination and strength needed to grab the lever and push the door out in the same motion was a challenge, so I made it one of my goals to accomplish.

Once I was inside I could use an elevator or walk down about twenty steps leading into the gym. I never used the elevator coming in or leaving for the entire two and a half years I attended the gym.

The light at the end of the tunnel seemed to be growing brighter. I had so much hope for my future. I was now able to reach high over my head to grab things. My legs and knees felt powerful. Having access to the gym was the key to a great deal of the improvement I reached.

My progress was the result of my continuous exercise and weight training, minus the thoughts of time running out. The only cost was my time and a small amount of money from my pocket. I was glad I did not have to worry about costs that could have been incurred by an insurance provider. I also realized that working out was without time restriction, opposite that of a rehabilitation institute or imposed by an insurance provider. Nonetheless, I am grateful for them both and the help they provided.

Chapter 8
A Showdown with Stroke #3
A Medical System in Reverse

Over the next few years, I regained my life. I had a son in 2004. My life was filled with satisfaction. Kim started working the graveyard shift after having the baby, and three months off from the job. My nights were spent feeding my son every two hours and changing pampers. After a year or so passed, my son and I began to ride everywhere and do everything together. In the coming years we spent several days at the park, Chucky Cheese, restaurants and the grocery store. Other times we spent time on the computer, cleaning the house, walking the block and waiting for mom to come home from work.

As the years passed, life was back to normal and I was beginning to use my left hand and arm more. I could turn corners while driving with my left hand. I was able to turn on the single lights in the S.U.V. or car. I could open doors, wash the car and other things with my left hand. It was not as strong as before and there were times I forgot to use it as much as I should have, but I was still able to use it when I purposely made the attempt.

I still had a left side limp but I had not used a cane in years. My son and I would go grocery shopping and would sometimes come home with over twenty bags. As little as he was, he would be the first to grab the bags. We had six steps to climb before getting inside the house, but we always had fun doing it.

On February 16, 2009, while driving home one night, I began to feel a tingling sensation in my right foot. I thought it was going *to sleep* on me so I continued to drive. Then I felt a numbing sensation in my right leg. I decided to keep driving since I was not too far from home. I drove along the streets where there was no traffic. I began driving very slow because I wanted to make sure I could stop. I pulled over once and decided to keep going. The time was about two a.m. I had about three blocks more before I would be at home.

Once I made it home I attempted to get out of the car, but I was too weak to stand. Using my cell phone, I called Kim who was inside the house. I told her I was outside and explained what was happening. She called an ambulance. I was taken to Memorial Hospital in Belleville, Illinois.

This time, I had right side weakness in my arm and leg but they were functional. I could talk very well and did not feel any other discomfort. From my past experiences, I knew I was having a stroke even though I was able to move my limbs.

By now, through my studies and experiences, I knew if you are experiencing stroke symptoms and if diagnosed and treated within a few crucial hours after symptoms appear, it might prevent further problems.

I inquired about the MRI and CT scan that could be done. The person on duty in the E.R. said they could run an MRI but if it did not show anything then they could not do a CT scan because they did not have the equipment. I inquired about the clot buster drug and the medical person said, if the MRI showed a blood clot then the medication to be used had a risk factor of a 50% chance of death and he did not advise this alternative.

After sitting in the emergency treatment room four hours with absolutely nothing being done, I felt like I was on a wait-to-see list. Even though nothing was being done by the staff, I had the feeling that at least I was in the right place if things became worse.

Kim and my daughter Tyan, who came to the hospital, remained with me for four hours, from 3 a.m. to 7 a.m. During those hours I was able to talk to them without any noticeable side effects. I never tried to stand up but I could move both legs and both arms. I did not know it for sure, but I believed at the time that I would be released to go home soon.

While lying in the emergency cubicle for hours, the only hospital staff that came to my area was those who ventured in and out to retrieve supplies from the cabinet. After not seeing or talking to anyone for the next few hours, I was finally told that I would be admitted to a room at 8 a.m. At that time Kim and Tyan decided to leave.

After being taken to a room in a wheelchair I was left alone for the next staff person to come. Around 8:30 a.m. a nurse came in and started asking me about my medical history. After she finished, she told me that she would be back shortly. I sat at a table in a wheelchair and waited. I watched the clock and about twenty minutes passed. During that time I started to feel a numbing sensation in my face.

The nurse returned to the room with a laptop and began asking me more medical questions. I tried to respond but this time my pronunciation was becoming slurred and talking became increasingly difficult. I told her that something was happening and I needed help. She said there were more questions she needed me to answer. I told her again that I needed help, and asked her to please call someone. I told her that I did not know what was going on, but I was having a hard time talking, and it felt like my face was going numb. I reminded her moments ago I was talking normally. I said, "Don't you remember that I was talking fine a while ago? Can't you hear the change in my voice? Please, call someone," I begged the nurse, but she continued to disregard what I said, and instead insisted that we finish the questions.

It was apparent to me that there was no way she could have known the first signs or symptoms of someone having a stroke. It was obvious because she totally disregarded my complaints about numbness in my face and difficulty with speaking. This should have been enough for her to react instead of being concerned with finishing a questionnaire. Furthermore, she should have noticed my slurred speech, but she did not. She acted like her main concern was completing her job assignment first and had no regard for the patient's health.

After going back and forth with the nurse, she paged the doctor on duty. She informed me that he was on his way to the hospital. She then said rather nonchalantly, 'let's get back to these questions'. Again, I tried to make her understand that something was affecting my body and I needed her to get another doctor or nurse. She said the doctor said he was about twenty minutes away and there was nothing she could do until he arrived.

When the doctor arrived he began to assess my situation. I detected displeasure in his voice towards the nurse that had paged him. I was immediately given some medication from his pocket and things started to get a little better. He scheduled an MRI. Before the MRI was complete, I had to be taken out of the machine to vomit on two separate occasions because of the medication I had received. After the second time, I was told to try to go through the MRI exam again. If I started to get nauseated again, they wanted me to show extra movement in my limbs, and they would immediately remove me from the MRI machine. They assured me that they would pay close attention and they did. For a third time, I became nauseated and started vomiting, so they removed me from the machine. The doctor requested something to settle my stomach. Quite a time passed but the medication did not come. My concern was to finish the MRI. Too much time had been wasted already, and I only had about a third of the way to go to complete the MRI, so I told the technicians that I would try to make it through the remainder of the exam. I was desperate to learn what had happened to me.

The results of the MRI revealed there was a blockage of an artery on the left side of my brain which affected the right side of my body.

I did not know what the next step was supposed to be, but I did expect more to happen medically. After the diagnosis was completed, I was taken to the same room and put to bed. For some reason I expected the doctor to return, and I also thought that I would receive some type of medication, but nothing happened. I saw no one until Kim and her sister showed, between noon and 1 o'clock p.m. After sitting a while, they also noticed that no hospital staff had come to my room. They asked me about it. I told them no one had been in to check on me or to say anything. Kim's sister went to ask the nurse why no one had checked in on me. The nurse told her they had called my family physician and they were waiting on him to get back with them. His office was in the building next door.

Kim and her sister sat with me for a while longer and finally asked me if I wanted to be transferred to Barnes Jewish Hospital in St. Louis because no one seemed to care if I received proper care or not. I immediately agreed to be transferred to Barnes.

Kim talked to one of the nurses about an ambulance to transfer me to Barnes before talking to my doctor about releasing me from the hospital, something he did not agree with me doing.

Kim decided to avoid confrontation with the doctor by deciding to call the ambulance service on her own. Without the doctor's referral, the ambulance trip would cost $899 cash. Kim was livid. She went to the doctor's office and screamed and carried on until he agreed to sign the release.

When my doctor came to sign the release, I did not see him. Kim told me that he had people in the waiting area of his office and probably did not have the time to stop by to see me before my transfer. However, while I was being wheeled to the ambulance I saw him passing by the elevator. When he saw me he asked me what happened. Initially, I could not understand why he asked me such a question. I was sure that Kim had explained to him why I wanted to be transferred, or the hospital staff should have told him. But I answered him anyway. "I think I had a stroke," I said. He touched me on the shoulder in a sympathetic way before he went on his way.

Afterwards I thought about some events of the past that happened between me and this doctor. During one of my quarterly visits to his office, he talked to me about the results of my blood work. Although my actual chart was not on his desk for him to refer to, he told me that my blood work showed a good reading. Everything he said sounded real good. It was exactly what any patient wants to here. What began to bother me as I thought about what he said was I was not aware of having blood work done prior to this particular visit.

I had been seeing this doctor for years. In the past, every visit that required blood work was followed up by a call from one of the nurse's aides from his office. They called to remind me that my doctor's appointment would be postponed if I had not had my blood work done. They wanted to make sure that the blood work from the lab was at his office in time for my visit.

Therefore, when he began telling me about my blood test results, I was confused and speechless, so I did not respond or question him. I did wonder how he could know test results from blood work that had not been performed. How can a doctor be trusted after telling his patient that all is well when no test had been done on my end, and no results had been turned in to his office, yet he said everything was fine? Several reasons for him doing what he did raced through my mind. Maybe he thought my files had been misplaced, and figured it would be better to fake a reading instead of admitting that the file could not be found. Perhaps he thought by telling me everything checked out okay, I would not give any thought to the fact that he had no file on his desk to read from. Apparently he failed to realize that having the chart or not, to read from, would not make a difference one way or the other because no blood work had been done. However, maybe it was easy for him to do because all he was concerned about was insuring that he received a payment from Medicare.

His actions made me think about the real intent of some doctors, especially when something like what he did occurred. He basically faked a medical reading. I believe what he did was a calculated decision that he made before I entered his treatment area.

If he had only been truthful and admitted that my paperwork had been misplaced, I could have alleviated some of his fears by telling him that no blood work had been done, so there would be no paperwork for blood test results. His failure to be truthful caused me to say nothing. Also at every blood chart reading, the Hepatitis C reading showed up, and he would inquire about the medical treatment from the gastrointestinal specialist he had referred me to visit. This time, he did not mention it.

The gastrointestinal specialist was located in the same building. We discussed treatment plans for my Hepatitis C. He sent me to Memorial Hospital for a colonoscopy, which was performed as outpatient surgery. The results of the colonoscopy checked out fine.

Months later the gastrointestinal specialist scheduled me to have an outpatient scope done on my esophagus. The results of this procedure also turned up fine. While I was in recovery after the esophagus procedure, Kim waited in the recovery room with me along with a technician from the hospital, who began going through a chart of questions.

One of the questions asked was, "How long have you had a problem with your throat?" To this question my first look was to Kim. We smiled at each other and I answered, "I have never had a problem with my throat." The technician must have seen the weird look on my face because she explained, "I asked because it's checked here that the patient said they had throat problems in the past." I responded by informing the technician that I had no idea where that information came from because I was never asked that question. I had no idea why I had been scheduled for this procedure anyway, but like many of us, we go along with the doctor's program and ask questions later. Because the doctor scheduled it, I figured it was okay. During my first office visit with this doctor, we talked about treatment for my Hepatitis C. After that, he scheduled me for two outpatient procedures. Each notification of the appointment was sent through the mail, not from an office visit. I figured they both had something to do with my Hepatitis C.

My primary doctor happened to be Kim's doctor too. Like he did me, he recommended that Kim go to the same doctor, who scheduled her for a colonoscopy as well. She was told that during her procedure he removed a polyp about the size of a golf ball, and that she needed to make a follow up visit in one year.

I also need to mention another incident with the primary doctor and Kim. She went in to have some tests done on her chest. He recommended Kim to go see an associate of his who was located in the same building as his office. After they looked at her chest x-ray results, Kim was called at home. The doctor insisted that she come to his office immediately. When she arrived, she was told that the x-rays showed spots on her lungs. She was immediately admitted to Memorial Hospital.

Kim spent five days as a patient, and during that time she racked up a hospital bill out of this world, only to find out the spots on the x-ray were not spots at all. But the hospital bill still had to be paid by her insurance provider, and she was left with an enormous deductible to pay.

It became quite obvious to me that our primary physician, on at least three occasions, passed information concerning his patients' problems on to his associates. My concern about this is how many other patients have gone through this or something similar? And my next question is why?

I am not suggesting that all practicing physicians treat their patients in this manner. I have to believe that many are truly passionate and sincere about the responsibilities and duties of their profession, and toward their patients, regardless of the situation. But there are enough negative viewpoints about the medical profession to imply that everything is not all right. It is true, that some people have spent a great portion of their life with the same physician without experiencing any discontent. And there are times when people have had the same doctor for years and once he was put to the real test of doing the right thing, something happened.

I suggest if you are disappointed in your doctor, ask for your records, and find another physician. Do not wait until things get bad.

Some physicians are faced with excessive financial obligations. Like so many of us, they are simply trying to make a decent living, but at what cost? We are the innocent, often trusting patients who rely on their professional, medical advice. We depend on their every suggestion of how to stay healthy and alive.

The afternoon of my third stroke, I was taken to Barnes Jewish Hospital and given an I.V. for the first time. I was feeling pretty bad at this time. All I could do was think back to the emergency room visit at Memorial Hospital in Belleville Illinois. I sat in Memorial Hospital for over seven hours without medical acknowledgement or assistance. It was there that I felt the wrath of my third stroke. It was there that I became totally disabled.

By the time I arrived at Barnes Jewish Hospital, I was totally disabled in both legs and arms. My chest felt like it was literally being squeezed with a metal band; and I could not take a full breath. A few times the pressure on my chest became so severe I could only scream. There was no pain, but the pressure was unbearable. I did not believe that anyone could do anything to make it better. While I was in the emergency room at Barnes Jewish Hospital, some of my family and friends came. I was in pretty bad shape, but I tried to show a measure of hope. To be truthful, I felt so many agonizing feelings that I actually believed I would be dead before the next day; and I had made peace with it.

While lying on the emergency room bed, I could not help thinking about many *what ifs* and *whys* leading up to my third debilitating stroke.

Why didn't Memorial Hospital perform an MRI when I first arrived? Was it because of the cost? *Why* did the emergency room staff mention an MRI to me but did not follow through with doing one? Was there proper staff on duty to perform the task? *What if* the MRI had been done when I first arrived and inquired about it? With all the obvious symptoms of a stroke, *why* did I have to be the one to ask about a procedure that should have been part of hospital protocol? If I had only been diagnosed sooner, I could have received proper care probably in time to prevent some of the trauma that came later. *Why? Why? Why?*

What if someone had been on staff to make better decisions that Sunday night? *Why* didn't they page the on call doctor for expert advice?

What if I had been put in ICU instead of a regular room at Memorial Hospital where closer medical care could have been given to me by better trained medical professionals? Was it because of the type of insurance coverage I had?

Why wasn't the medical person who questioned me about my medical history more educated about common symptoms of a stroke? – Facial, arm, or leg weakness; problems with speech.

What happens when your primary care physician is too busy for you in an emergency? Was he too busy to inquire about my symptoms, and give advice over the phone? Didn't he have the ability to check his patient's medical history and relay some type of treatment to the hospital for stabilization?

Looking back over everything that transpired, I can say without a moment's hesitation that my life and that of my family have been terribly disrupted.

At the time of writing this book, over eight years has passed since my second stroke, and over two years has passed since my third stroke, and I am still suffering from that night. I cannot take out the trash; I can barely attach the bag to the trash can. All of which used to be simple acts that I used to take for granted and could do without effort. These simple tasks are the same things that I can no longer do and maybe never do again. I have been living with weakness to my left side for years but driving, walking, slow running and moving large furniture still had not been a problem for me – until that fateful night.

After the seven-hour window came and went without receiving treatment at Memorial Hospital, and with no concern for my well-being, I could very easily be sentenced to spend the rest of my life in a nursing facility. I know this was not a one-of-a-kind incident for a hospital or the first time this type of situation occurred at this hospital. There must have been others in the past and there will be more people put in this helpless situation in the future and no one will ever understand why. With the hundreds of thousands of disabled people at home and in the nation home care facilities, and with me experiencing this, it makes me wonder how some of those people got there.

Understaffed and overworked, are some words that spring to mind for me from my 2:30 a.m. Monday morning visit in the emergency room at Memorial Hospital of Belleville Illinois. Why don't these people realize, the health care service is not there to just provide them with an opportunity to have a job or a top position, but to get the patients better. It may seem a bit naive to expect this but at least a little common sense should enter into this. How many patients, have been wrongly diagnosed, or have not been diagnosed at all, because an over worked person was expected to work long hours, or expected to contact the on call Doctor when they are not sure whether the situation is important enough.

I can tell you right now, today, on Saturday 10:35 pm Christmas day December 25, 2010 while sitting at home not having the ability or desire to visit my family or friends, then I'd say on that particular night at Memorial Hospital, the decision to call that on call doctor at 3:00am instead of 9:30 a.m. could have made a big difference in my life, my son's life and my family's life. Not being able to go outside yesterday to play with my son in the snow like last year, or assist him in opening his Christmas gifts this morning like before, then I think the situation was important enough to call or page the on call doctor.

I have no doubts that it was financially beneficial in the short term for the hospital to have a doctor on staff and who knows where with a pager but what about the patient's care and real decisions being made by the inexperienced medical staff standing around watching the clock early into the mornings. In order for that on call doctor to be fully functional in making crucial life sustaining decisions, someone who cannot make that decision is in charge of calling the doctor.

We are all vulnerable where a stroke is concerned, no matter what age. The impact is devastating both for the survivor and their families. A stroke may leave you with paralysis of one side of the body causing visual and or cognitive problems or muscle weakness on one side of the body causing disablement. A stroke occurs when a blood vessel in the brain is blocked or bursts. Without blood and the oxygen it carries, part of the brain starts to die. The part of the body controlled by the damaged area of the brain cannot work properly.

Brain damage can set in within minutes, so it is important to know the symptoms of stroke and act fast. Quick treatment can help limit damage to the brain and increase the chance of a full recovery.

You need to see a doctor right away. If a stroke is diagnosed immediately after symptoms begin, doctors may be able to use medicines that can help you recover.

The first thing the doctor needs to find out is what kind of stroke it is: ischemic or hemorrhagic. This is important because the medicine given to treat a stroke caused by a blood clot could be deadly if used for a stroke caused by bleeding in the brain.

To find out what kind of stroke it is, the doctor will do a type of X-ray called a Ct scan of the brain, which can show if there is bleeding. The doctor may order other tests to find the location of the clot or bleeding, check for the amount of brain damage, and check for other conditions that can cause symptoms similar to a stroke.

At 2:30 a.m. when I first arrived at Memorial Hospital I was taken straight into an emergency treatment room with all signs of a stroke. Why did the on call doctor not send me immediately for an MRI which would have shown a blocked artery or eliminated that possibility? Was it that he had not been contacted or he had to weigh whether to waste money on the MRI and have it come back normal? Or was it that they do not have that facility open on weekends, because of the overtime. Surely the powers that be know that you can get ill on the weekend. I apologize if I'm getting carried away, but I have suffered and I am still suffering mentally and physically a great deal every day. I have a tremendous disability because there were too many non-decision makers working at a major city hospital on a Sunday night...

After transferring from Memorial Hospital in Illinois to Barnes Jewish Hospital in Missouri and after treatment, I was taken to Barnes Rehabilitation Institute.

The third stroke brought on right side paralysis and affected the previous stroke on the left side and paralyzed my left arm and leg. This caused me to lose all ability to stand or walk on both limbs and also the loss of use of both arms.

The therapy was scheduled to begin a week later on February 23, 2009. The only thing I have to say after lying in bed and looking around at the walls and hearing the sounds coming from the hallway and the noises from other patients in other rooms, are a few four word comments. Isn't this a B.? What have I done? I cannot believe this. I was going through a feeling like I was repeating my worst nightmare. I remembered the promise I had made to myself six years ago. I said, I never wanted to forget this miserable feeling and I needed to do whatever it takes to avoid putting myself through an ordeal like this ever again. I guess my head did not get bumped hard enough the last time. I think the bump on my head is about a foot long now because I feel as though I was hit with a sledge hammer this time.

Here I am again. I am just lying here. I cannot even scoot my body over. I cannot adjust the pillow under my head. I cannot reach and grab the cover to cover my arms. My face feels as though I am standing in front of a heat vent. I am constantly feeling like the furnace is turned up too high but my body is cold to the touch. I cannot wash my face. I can barely hold a spoon or find my mouth with the spoon. My mind is aware of everything but my body is like a disconnected refrigerator. Nothing is working. My thinking and memory are very clear and I can understand everything that's going on around me. I know what's coming next and what is expected of me but, I wish I could go back to sleep and wake up and this nightmare was over.

During the week before the physical therapy began, each day was spent assessing how well I could manage things like eating, washing, remembering things etc. To be honest I never imagined there was a worse feeling than the second stroke but this time I felt as though the second stroke was simple to deal with in comparison to what I am feeling now. The only things I can do well are talk and remember.

I created a happy state of mind but I was miserable. I wanted so badly for the therapy to start so I could begin trying to weather this storm. I had all the confidence in the world that once physical and occupational therapy began the days would begin to clear up for me.

Once therapy started for me, I just knew things would be looking up. But during the first week of therapy I began to sense that my treatment was not going well. I liked the therapist because she was a very serious worker, but she seemed to be a little distracted. She seemed from the first session to be confident and sure of her every move. She probably did not know at the time that I had high hopes and all the confidence in the world that recovery was on its way. I was in bad shape but I was observing and analyzing everything being done.

In the beginning I did not give much thought to it but now I have to figure that the therapist was under extra pressure because the stroke had actually altered both sides of my body. The pressure of having to give therapy to a patient with no ability to walk on either limb and also to someone that could hardly hold on to a crutch, had to weigh heavy on her mind. Also, there is the possibility that the insurance was covering physical therapy for the right side and not the left side and being that the recent stroke caused right side disability but completely paralyzed the left side also, created a major problem for the therapist and possibly for the facility.

My knowing that this was a rehabilitation institute; my question is where are the experts? If not for physical help then where were they for advice? The therapist at times seemed to have a direct plan and if it did not work immediately, she would decide on something else. At this time I was weak but ready to work as hard as possible. I had no problem with hard work because I knew what was required of me. As bad as I felt I did not and would not for one second let things gets me down.

Each day I would say I plan on being able to walk when I'm released. I actually did not know for sure but I knew I was ready to work at it.

As the days and weeks began to pass, I began to since that very little progress was being made. I was still walking like the scarecrow on the Wizard of Oz. I could stand and walk a little with the walker along with the therapist's support but I could not let go nor could the therapist let me go for one second without a fall. Regardless of how much walking support I had, my legs would only carry me so many feet before they would completely collapse. The therapist would try letting me stand with the hemi-cane which has lots of support for the average stroke victim but I had absolutely no balance for even one second of standing alone. She tried strapping me in two different full body machines and neither gave her the response she was looking for.

As the days continued to pass I could since the therapist trying but did not seem to have an answer. Even though I was in really bad shape there was never a team effort like I had experienced years before. I guess there were no experts on my situation to consult with or to assist. The therapist seemed to be confused on what treatment to do. Nothing was consistent. As more time passed I began to feel as though things weren't going to well but I was still with hope and determination. As hard as I was prepared to work I was very weak and could only rely on the next step taken by the therapist. I guess I was not focused enough to ask, do you need help or is there someone else that we can consult with for more information on my condition? Plus I did not realize time was running out.

After you deal with one stroke, you will need a lot of motivation to deal with the affects of another and especially if your condition is worse than before. I honestly did not believe the third stroke which was to my right side was as bad as the second, but because of not recovering full usage of my left arm and leg from before, the third stroke affected my left side to the point of rendering it totally lifeless. My left arm and leg could not move at all.

At the start of the fourth week of therapy, my case worker said I would probably be released to go home or to a nursing facility because my insurance would not agree to more inpatient therapy. She said if my choice was to go home, then I would need an access ramp built. I immediately got in touch with a carpenter friend and made arrangements for a ramp to be built.

The day before my release the therapist from occupational therapy took me upstairs to a large exercise equipment room and asked if I wanted to work out on any of the equipment. I did not know this room existed. For the first time I got to work out on a leg press, and the feeling was great. Kim was with me and I told her how good it felt and now I wish I had more time.

This was one of the key components missing from my therapy routine everyday, which possibly would have benefited me weeks earlier, along with the walking and standing exercise I did receive.

For the entire four weeks of inpatient therapy I did not receive any direct exercise at all to create any muscles. There was an exercise bike just feet away but I thought sooner or later I would get to use it. More exercise could have increased the evaluation at the end of four weeks and may have been enough to recommend additional weeks of therapy.

I guess I was too caught up in my illness to realize the treatment could have improved and the therapist was possibly under a lot of pressure. I cannot dismiss the thought that being under the umbrella of Medicare /Medicaid insurance this time, may have played a large part in the amount of treatment I could receive. I guess my thoughts are in this direction because of so many other times I had been confronted with the situation that I was not as important of a person anymore because of having government insurance. When someone would say, we do not accept Medicaid Medicare insurance then I would just move on. Or when a medical facility would say we cannot take you because we are not 100% sure we will be paid. All this time I was trying to get my disability together and I did not give enough thought to the change of acceptance by the medical community. I refuse to believe society's people have changed this drastically so I have to put the blame on the different insurance I have at this time. The possibilities of extensive therapy did not exist this time and I was not in any condition to question these decisions.

I was back at the same facility as before but things felt so different this time. It seemed as though the attitude of the medical people had changed, and with that change the quality of service had changed.

One example of the feeling of a change is the

physical therapist was prompt every time on every thirty minute session, but the occupational therapist was late on an average of ten minutes on every three out of five sessions and because of other patients waiting; the time could not be made up.

One day the occupational therapist was late and at the end of my session, she saw that I was free for the next thirty minutes and asked if I wanted to stay even though she had another patient. My answer was if I can get more therapy then yes. She went and picked up her next patient and she had both of us at the same table for treatment for which I did not mind because I was getting additional therapy treatment. During the treatment for the two of us together she was up and gone so many times that there was still only about fifteen minutes of therapy actually done. I also saw her work sheet where she had left it on the table and my name was marked down for two therapy sessions and one session for the other patient. Like I said before my mind was clear and I was aware of everything going on around me. I guess anyone seeing how bad my physical condition was would have a misconception of my thinking ability. During the therapy sessions with me feeling so bad I just did not have a lot to talk about so only a few people knew there was nothing wrong with my mental state. I think if she had known this she would have taken her therapy schedule with her.

The very next day she was late again and asked again did I want to stay the next thirty minutes. The wheelchair I was using was very uncomfortable, and I could feel the metal frame. It had my bottom and my back so uncomfortable, all I could think about was getting a break from the chair. As much as I wanted the opportunity to have extra therapy I told her I could not stay. She insisted that I stay but I was not having it. After taking me back to my room, she attempted to leave me in the middle of the floor, as if she was in a hurry to get back. The therapist knew I was not able to transfer from the wheelchair to the bed and normally they would assist you to bed. I had to call out in a raised voice to get her to help me from the chair to the bed. She seemed very agitated, but I surely did not care because, none of this would be happening if she had been on time in the first place.

At the beginning of the second week, I thought the therapist would be more prompt. If I had been able I would have wheeled myself to therapy on time everyday but because I was too weak I had to wait on her.

After voicing my concerns of losing treatment time to the doctor in charge of the facility, the therapy supervisor came to my room. Actually, this lady whose name I will not mention, had talked with me when I first arrived because we remembered each other from years before. She was the therapist working with me the day I spoke about the guy who was drenched in sweat. She was one of three therapist I saw, still there from six years ago.

One morning just before the session in question, the supervisor came to my room to hear what I had to say. After hearing me she realized that I was concerned about losing time in therapy and she complemented me on that because as she said there are so many patients who need motivation and lots of encouragement to do therapy.

I did not think about it then but I guess she planned to see me at that time to see firsthand for herself about my complaint. While we were talking, the time came for my treatment with the therapist in question. She arrived as usual, ten minutes late. She peeped into the room and saw her supervisor and said she would be right back. I guess she thought when she came back her supervisor would be gone and she could make up her time for being late by keeping me an additional thirty minutes. When the therapist finally came back, her supervisor was still there and it was plain to see that I only had ten minutes left on my therapy session. The next morning she was taken off of my case.

After the first occupational therapist was removed for being late so often, then her replacement showed. Well like the old saying goes, sometimes you cannot win for losing. The next one was as bad as the first. This time I could not get a good working person to help me in my recovery. I was ready and willing to do whatever it took to get my body to the next level whatever it would be and with no complaints. But the problem was getting the therapist to cooperate.

The new occupational therapist took three days of my sessions making a splint for my left wrist. The reason she took so long was because she kept screwing up and starting over. For the entire thirty minutes I just sat there watching. My first thoughts were that she would make me a nice splint. After the second day my good thoughts were beginning to fade. I thought about years ago there was a splint making facility a few blocks from the Institute. I knew this because before I left the facility in 2003, the company had made a leg splint and an arm splint for me and I went to pick them up myself. Maybe this was a way of saving money but, just give this some thought. For each of the three days of attempting to make a splint, the institution and the therapist billed the insurance provider for therapy time that I never received. And by the way, the splint never got made because the therapist gave up.

Two days later my therapist showed up accompanied by a student who was present during my therapy sessions. All I did during the following two days was answering an endless list of questions. At this time I was completing the second week in therapy and my inpatient treatment days were about to end. I actually felt no amount of improvement in the time I had spent at the facility. I knew if I didn't show some type of progress I would be denied additional treatment.

Another prime example of the change in the quality of health care I received was, because of my restriction to the bed, I had to buzz for assistance. There were some nights I would wake up to discover that my urinal was unusable. One night I could not wait for the assistant to come and change my urinal, so I was forced to double use it. Of course, because of my stroke, my steadiness was not that great. I wasted urine in the bed. This situation made me feel humiliated, angry, helpless and useless. Here I was, a grown man, lying in my own urine and there was nothing I could do but wait for someone to come to my room and clean me up. Having to be cleaned like a baby was devastating. I even wondered if the nursing assistant may have thought I had lied about wasting the urinal. After all, they did not know anything about me, my medical condition or whether I was one who actually wetted the bed, like my roommate who had to be cleaned twice every night.

After that terrible, dehumanizing mishap, I began buzzing for an assistant several times on a single occasion to empty my urinal. I did not want to chance falling asleep, only to wake up with a full urinal and bladder – a deadly combination. Most of the time about forty-five to sixty minutes passed before an assistant arrived so I had to change my strategy. I started calling for a urinal change as soon as I recognized that my urinal had not been serviced. Sometimes the urinal was returned by the assistant without being rinsed.

There were plenty of things I could have easily complained about, but some of the technicians came to work with negative attitudes. I saw things that I did not agree with, but I felt it would not be proper to complain to the staff because they were the very ones I had to depend on for care.

The early shift usually had better staff, but when the evening shift arrived, I could count good working technicians on two fingers. It was probably because they were tired and irritable because they had to pull a double shift.

Thinking about things later, I recall that the last time I was at this rehabilitation institution, the room I occupied was a couple of doors away, and on the opposite side from two double doors which remained locked around the clock. Any time someone entered or left this area, they either used a code or had to be buzzed in and out.

The atmosphere I was in on the inside of these locked double doors was that of a facility whose patients were mentally unstable or in need of special nursing home type care. I often heard patients screaming out loud which further substantiated my thoughts about the facility. I thought the patients had suffered a stroke but there was also something about some of them that seemed odd. For instance, there was one patient that wondered the hall constantly and set off the alarm at the door. At night while my lights were out he would come into my room talking loud in a crazy way about hurting someone. I would have to call for a staff member to remove him. Every time someone came to get him they would tell me, 'Oh, he's harmless', like that was supposed to make me feel better.

There was one technician I happened to know. We were from the same home town. He often talked about the mental condition of his patients. He said there were times he had to clean feces from the floor because some of them walked around naked and freely defecated.

On the other side of the double doors was a much different atmosphere. It was where my room was six years ago when I had my second stroke. I may be wrong and hopefully, I am; but the last time I was at this facility I had private insurance through the job. This time around, I have government insurance which leaves me wondering about this and many other unexplainable events relating to my care, or lack thereof. For example, it was apparent that I was not properly attended to when I was at Memorial Hospital.

Months later after being at home, I began to take notice and watch documentaries and television specials about the poor quality of patient care in many hospitals, and nursing homes. Watching these reports was like watching someone who was describing the life I had lived. I listened to stroke victims and their caregivers reveal their frustration about the total lack of quality patient care administered by many facilities and the poor services received from institutions around the country.

Complaints about mistakes and delays in receiving

medical treatment were often talked about. Some patients told of being treated like they were stupid; while other former patients talked about not being fed, not being taken to or from the toilet on time, and going several days without a bath.

There were also reports of stroke victims who were not treated in hospital wards intended for that purpose, but were instead placed and left in psychiatric units...

Patients who were treated in the appropriate stroke units praised their level of care, but those in general wards were often the ones who experienced poor treatment such as not being given prompt and adequate access to vital services like physical therapy or speech therapy.

Patients who were unable to speak were not washed, and went without water because they could not communicate. Upon being discharged, stroke victims felt they were left to cope alone without adequate resources, knowledge, or support.

Coming across this information after having experienced the same things they spoke about, I could only sit and listen in disbelief, knowing from firsthand experience that their stories were not tall tales. To know this kind of inhumane and unfair treatment of human beings existed in this country in many patient care facilities is probably difficult for the average, healthy, well-insured person to believe.

In the past, I recall seeing on various occasions on the evening news reports about abuse in home care facilities. When the news went off, I must sadly admit, so did my thoughts about the abuse. Now I understand that the patients who live under these conditions cannot turn from one channel to the next, or turn the television on or off to make their suffering go away.

Think about it, the patient affected by such abuse lives in that facility but because a person is in bad physical shape, they should not be treated like they cannot feel mental and physical abuse. Living in these conditions can only make a person worse off, knowing they have to put up with this every day without a way of escape. There are thousands of patients affected in verbal, physical, and neglectful ways by medical staff members; and quite often, after a short time, these patients do take a turn for the worse.

I witnessed an elderly male patient, when I was at one of these facilities, who became upset with one of the technicians at the nursing home. Probably at first thought, anyone passing the scene of the loud disturbance looked at the man as being out of order or out of control. It appeared that no one actually stopped and thought that he had become fed up with the way he was being treated and was justified for the anger he displayed.

As I mentioned earlier, when I arrived at the institute after my third stroke, my body was close to being a total wreck, and my speech was somewhat impaired, but my thoughts were clear and aware. My guess is that the medical personnel, after assessing my physical condition, assumed that my mind was just as bad. The attitude of some of the staff was unbelievable and no one in charge said or did anything about it. I witnessed the same uncaring attitudes from the staff when I used to visit my mother at the nursing home. It was not towards my mother while I was there, but I definitely saw other residents at that nursing home whose level of treatment was totally out of order.

My condition was high risk for falling so I was not able to leave the bed without assistance. Getting a toilet assistant was like pulling teeth. After a bowel movement I had to wait thirty minutes for an assistant to return. Even after pushing the call button several times while I sat on the stool.

I can understand that medical personnel can be extremely busy at times, but what if I was pushing the bathroom call button because I had fallen and there was a real emergency? Think about how long I, or another patient, would have been lying on the floor before being rescued.

One of the better working technicians came to assist me from the toilet one evening. She was angry because as she said, "I do not get paid for toilet assisting. They need to get rid of some of these workers."

Most of the technicians worked twelve hour shifts. Some technicians were requested to work a double shift and were probably exhausted. This can cause employees to avoid certain work and even hide and take mini sleep breaks.

"Complaints are nothing new around here. The technician for this call is right out there in the hall and heard the switchboard calling her name, but she just avoided the call," she told me.

On another occasion, there was a technician who was assisting me from the toilet. She asked for help from another tech who happened to be standing by her. The two of them were talking casually at the time. Instead of helping her, she walked away.

The technician said, "Now I know that bitch heard me ask her for help, and she deliberately walked off."

One night, my urinal needed to be emptied. I told

my roommate that I was going to buzz for the technician and see how long it would take before someone responded. In an hour's time, I buzzed six times. All six times the switchboard answered. She only called out over the intercom for a technician two out of those six times. One hour after the first buzz, someone finally came to my room. My roommate and I agreed that this situation was pitiful. After so much of this type of unprofessional treatment, I finally complained to the head nurse over the hospital wing.

Her solution: "Would it help if I ordered you an additional urinal?"

At the time it sounded like a reasonable idea so I said, "Yes." I figured it was the easier way to solve the issue so I had no problem with it. But later on, I started to think about what had occurred, and her suggestion was not for my benefit. I came to the conclusion that I was given an extra urinal, not for my needs, but as a means to cover up poor service and keep me quiet.

I am sure many of you know something about the terrible state of healthcare in our country. This is partially the fault of people in the healthcare industry who prey on the ill. They escalate healthcare costs, charge for services that are not performed, bring in extra help when it is not needed, perform unnecessary services at the time, and the list can go on and on.

There were occasions when people visited my room and asked me questions. Afterward they would give me the same advice that other medical personnel who came before them had already given me. Eventually I began to wonder who they were and why they were coming to see me. At first, I did not question the reasons for the visits because I assumed these individuals were part of the staff. Sometimes they would come in and pull up a chair and sit next to my bed and start with questions about my day. After they left I would ask myself, what was that all about?

After arriving home I started being billed for thirty-minute therapy sessions. I did not remember who the people were, and at a charge between $120 and $140, along with me being responsible for 50%, a revelation came to me. I had one word that summed it up—fraud.

Regardless of the type of insurance you have, whether it is private or government insurance, there are certain procedures that are much the same. After my private insurance coverage was dropped, I applied for Medicaid. Both private insurance and Medicaid require you to show a percentage of improvement after a certain amount of time, or other alternatives will be recommended.

My intention is not to scare you, but to open your eyes to *the realities of a stroke* and the system operating around you. I hope what I am sharing will help motivate you to work for better progress for yourself. If you are a patient, do not miss one minute of therapy. Next, learn exactly what you need to do. Remember, the therapist has a limited amount of time to work with you, and the insurance provider has a limited amount of money that will be put towards your recovery. Your cooperation and motivation are very important for your future recovery.

The success of your treatment may depend on you and the determination of the medical facility, to improve your condition in a certain amount of time. This is largely determined by a percentage of improvement based on and set forth by an earlier evaluation performed on you.

If, after weeks of treatment, you show a substantial percentage of improvement, then per request from the therapist and the medical facility to your doctor and/or insurance provider, you could possibly be granted additional weeks of therapy.

Chapter 9
Back Home After Stroke #3
Coping and Hoping

After my third stroke, I had a huge problem with walking, standing, and leaning from a chair, along with several other physical problems. This was because of the loss of strength, feeling and coordination on both sides of my body.

There existed a feeling of anger in me about the stroke, but I never let anyone know. This time, I had plenty of reasons to be worried about how well I would recover, but I never said a word. I never admitted it but I felt uncomfortable and embarrassed about the loss of everyday abilities that I was once able to do. There were days when I lost patience with myself for not being able to do certain things.

I had to face the fact that I looked terrible, and aside from that I felt terrible. To keep from going to a nursing home from the hospital, I lied to my case worker and said that I had a service ramp built at my home. I just wanted to get back home, at any cost. I knew that when a person in my condition is put into a nursing home, it would mean being restricted to a bed, and my physical condition would probably never improve.

After a stroke, there may be times when you feel an overwhelming sense of sadness about your disabilities, or you may be sad because you are uncertain about your future. You may even feel guilty about the stress; changes and hardships caused within your family that you believe are a result of your stroke. You might think that you could have done something to prevent it from happeningl. You might feel that you need to do more to help, and it angers you even more when you realize that you cannot. Sometimes your stroke can bring up guilt about events that took place in the past. You may feel alone or lonely, and at times believe that no one understands what you are going through. You may feel a need to talk about some of these feelings, but you wonder if you would really be heard or even if it would do any good if you were.

After going through four weeks of inpatient therapy at Barnes Rehabilitation Institute from February to March 23, 2009 for five days a week, I came home and had no improvement at all. I could not stand up for two seconds without grabbing on to something to hold myself up. I had no strength or balance in my legs.

My first day home I tried to use a walker. However, I had no idea that I was not ready for a walker. To try and make the walker move evenly, a crutch type extension was installed for my left arm to rest on. It was elevated about ten inches over my walker. Since I could not use my left arm, it kept me off balance while I attempted to use the walker. To help, a Velcro strap was attached to it in order to hold my arm on the walker for balance.

I must have walked about eight feet into the bedroom when I mistakenly flipped up the end of a throw rug. Instead of continuing to walk, my plan was to use the leg of the walker to press down the flipped end of the rug. I did not realize I had lifted the entire walker from the floor, and without it I had no ability to stand. Before I could say oops, I fell helplessly backwards still strapped to the walker.

I hit the back of my head on the corner of the

doorway. The impact was so hard I felt the back of my head to see if I was bleeding, but fortunately I was not. It hurt really badly, but not as much as realizing that I did not have enough strength to pull myself up to a crawling position so I could get to the chair.

Once I turned over onto my belly, I began making the motions to get up. My first attempt was unsuccessful, but I tried again. The problem was that my body, because of the muscles lost, seemed to weigh a ton and because of the weakness, I could not get my arms underneath to make an attempt for a lift. Once I maneuvered my hand in the right position, I struggled hard, but I soon realized my arms did not have enough power to do what was once a very simple task. My son, Kaden, who was five years old at the time, was there with me.

After he saw that I could not get up, he said, "Dad, I'm going to get Mom." He went next door for help where Kim was visiting her sister.

Not being able to get up from the floor really hurt my pride. Even though I knew I was in bad shape from the stroke, I never imagined there would ever come a time in my life when I could not get up from the floor. Believe me, when my son left to get help, I relentlessly tried to get up because I did not want anyone to see me helplessly lying in the floor. I was flat against the floor as if I was glued down. This was so unexpected and a huge blow to my ego. It really took a while to soak into my head that regardless of how strong my inner thoughts were about getting up, my body was unable to perform the task.

When help arrived, I was assisted to the wheelchair. Yet, sometimes even now, I honestly cannot believe after all of that unsuccessful struggling I did not get discouraged. Instead, I got pissed off. I do not know if it was because I could not get up from the floor or because of the weeks of therapy I had just completed, that seemed to amount to a big fat zero. That many weeks and hours of therapy should have shown at the least, a glimpse of light at the end of the tunnel. I knew the therapy at the institute had been lacking in accomplishments, but this made it seem like nothing at all had been done. I felt like I had just been chosen to be the fall guy in a big con job. If I had spent $31,000 for anything, which was the total bill for my stay in rehab, then you better believe I would definitely be expecting something in return.

The insurance company put the money up for services, the rehab institute and the therapists got the money for a job well planned but not done, and I was left holding an empty bag.

Even though it would have been an easy thing to do, I did not allow their lack of accomplishments at the rehabilitation center to affect my will to do things on my own. I understood that they had years of training and experience treating people with disabilities, yet I never thought for one second that I could not do a better job. With my determination and my tendency to succeed, I could and would do a better job on myself and for myself. I had to get better, so it was the same will and determination that overshadowed the fact that the experts had given up on me. Until now, I had never given any thought to the amount of influence the insurance provider had over my life. Regardless of the possibility that I might get better, they had thrown the towel in on me and I never realized it.

My immediate plan was to work on my arm strength, so the next time I fell I would be able to get up. It was not long before I fell again, a few weeks at the most. This time it was while going into the bathroom. Kim was at home. She came to help me get up. I told her to let me attempt to get up on my own, because I needed to know if I could do it myself. A few minutes later, slippery floor, cramped up area and all, I was the proudest man on earth because I got up into a standing position, holding on to the sink. Kim did not say anything but I knew it helped her confidence in me.

After the fall on my first day home, I decided I was not ready to use my walker, even though the therapist had me using it constantly during my final week of inpatient rehabilitation.

I had to immediately map out a plan for myself at home. I definitely did not want anyone worrying that something of that magnitude would happen again. Regardless of how safe you try to be, accidents will happen and for my sake, the safety of my son, and the confidence of my lady, I had to get control of my days.

I decided to call my friend, Derrick "G.I. Joe" Glover, whom I knew I could trust. G.I. Joe's father was also recovering from a stroke. He had been spending the early portions of his days at home with him, so he was already adapted to caring for someone with my type of disability. With someone helping me I could not walk ten feet without my legs collapsing; but I had plans to improve that slowly but surely.

When I contacted my friend, I asked him to come to my home Monday through Wednesday for two hours a day at $25 per day to assist me. I had only my disability income but I had to sacrifice some things. I could have asked if he could assist me for free, but that did not seem right. Even though I did not have much money, I was prepared to sacrifice.

I had to make this arrangement because I did not want to limit myself to what I had gone through the past four weeks. I figured, when the outpatient therapy started I would learn what to do and continue the routine at home.

I went into the hospital February 16, 2009 and came home on Thursday March 23, 2009. My personal home therapy was to begin on Monday March 27, 2009. My new doctor scheduled me for outpatient therapy at St. Elizabeth's on the following Monday April 4, 2009.

The first day of at-home therapy I had my friend to make a fist and hold his arm out as stiff as possible waist high like a cane. When I took two steps then he would do the same. I do not know how I came up with this plan; it just felt like the thing to do. The first day with him and my sister, Lillie, watching me, I was able to walk eight feet. My body was doing a terrible lean but I did it; and my sister was there on time with the wheelchair each time I stopped. I must have taken a twenty minute break and then I walked another ten feet. The third time, I managed to walk eight feet again, and I was done for the day. I was extremely tired and my legs were fatigued, but my sister, G.I. Joe, and I, were all on such a high because I was able to get on my feet and move, without someone holding me up with a belt. I basically felt like what I had achieved in a two hour span of time was more satisfying than anything I had done in the past four weeks. Finally, I felt like there was hope.

The second day went pretty much the same as the first day. On my third day of at home therapy, while using the wrist cane, I walked twelve feet and stood in front of the wheelchair for four seconds without any assistance. The second walk was twenty minutes later and I covered ten feet. The third walk was about twenty minutes later and I covered eighteen feet. This time I made it to the bedroom and turned around and said, "I'm going to walk back to the kitchen." Well, my legs had a different idea. Like two rubber bands hooked under my body, they began to collapse. G.I. Joe held me up and called for Lillie to bring my wheelchair. Needless to say, that was the end of that session for the day. Eventually, we started stationing a regular chair in certain parts of the house just in case my legs gave out again.

The following Monday was the first day of outpatient therapy. I was attempting to get to the car with the help of Kim. She had seen me at the rehab center almost every day, but she had not seen me one on one trying to get around without my wheelchair. Just seeing me struggling coming down the steps and trying to get into the car was all new to her. And to tell the truth, all of this was new to me too, because I had never walked down any steps unassisted since my last stroke. The only time I had attempted to get into a car was the day I left the rehabilitation center.

With Kim's help and I guess from her experiencing firsthand how much assistance I needed, she asked, "Do you think you'll ever walk again?"

I had no response to her question, because I really did not know what to say. While we were driving to the rehabilitation center, her question replayed over and over in my head. The thought of me not being able to walk on my own again had never entered my mind, because I was so focused on working as hard as possible to walk.

All of a sudden I began to feel like I was living in denial of the truth. During all this time, I had not taken the time to assess the damages the stroke had caused and whether or not it was fixable. I had never looked for an opinion from someone just observing me. I know that when people saw me in this condition they had their own opinions and thoughts about my future but had no reason to express it aloud, and especially to me. Most people would probably keep those thoughts to themselves if only to respect my feelings. I was so caught up in my expectations of walking again, that I never phantom the thought of whether it was possible or impossible. During the ride to the center, I became very depressed and then angry; but I managed to keep these feelings to myself because I knew Kim meant no harm in asking.

By the time we arrived at the rehabilitation center, my anger had turned into determination. I did begin to feel that Kim should not have questioned whether I would ever walk again, but in a way, I was glad she did because it became a motivator for me. At a later date in time, I reminded Kim of the question she'd asked me. I actually thanked her for being bold enough to say what was on her mind.

Every morning of outpatient therapy, even in the rain sometimes, I had to walk down six large concrete steps. There may have been only six steps but for me, it felt like twenty. While walking down the stairs I had to grab the railing but could not get a good grip, because my right hand was numb and weak. I felt like I was going down the side of a mountain without a lot of control. I was terrified, but I said nothing because it had to be done. All I could do was to keep saying over and over to myself, "The more times I do this, the better at it I'll become."

Going up the stairs was a strain, but not as fearful as going down the stairs.

After getting the opportunity to come home, I had a wonderful support team with me. When I came home, I was going through the most difficult period ever of my life, but I held on to my will and determination to get better. Plus, I felt more at ease because Kim had my back, my five-year old son kept my safety and parenting skills on the forefront, my sister, Lillie, provided her good cooking and support, my friend and hired assistant, G.I. Joe, along with my computer kept my mind busy. There were some cloudy days and the water was rough, but the storm of my life was being well-managed.

The first week of April 2009 was the beginning of my outpatient therapy. I had occupational and physical therapy three days a week during the first month, for forty-five minutes per session.

During therapy, I used a walker. I leaned terribly because of weakness in my joints and the fear of falling. Even though the therapist was holding me by a belt around my chest, I still felt unsteady because I had absolutely no balance or power. I could only maneuver the walker with one hand because my left arm was bent and stiff, and if I could get my hand to hold it, I would lift it off the floor. My right leg moved okay but slowly, while my left leg had hardly any lifting power.

I was determined, but I could not imagine what was in the future for me. I would force myself to walk twenty feet before resting. I would do about nine leg lifts and rest again and try to walk twenty more feet and do about twenty reps on the leg press equipment. I wanted to do more, but the therapists suggested that I should not do as much right now.

I asked the therapist about working more on my left leg. Her response was that she was not interested in my left leg; rather her therapy treatment was for my right leg. The answer was sort of confusing but I never asked for more clarification. I wondered if it was because of my insurance being directed towards my present stroke or if it was better to improve my right leg usage since it would be better to stabilize the stronger leg first?

The forty-five minute sessions were over so quickly that it felt as though the sessions lasted about fifteen minutes instead. My walking was so slow it took me fifteen minutes to cover twenty feet. An example of progress from then to now is that now I can cover three hundred feet in fifteen minutes.

The wheelchair was my best friend. It was very difficult getting around the house because of the carpet. My right arm and right leg were not very strong, but they were the best I had for operating the chair on the carpet. My left side had no function at all as far as movement. After three weeks of continuous and hard work at home and at the rehab center, I folded the wheelchair. I still used it every day outside the house for therapy and also doctors' visits. I had no intentions of going anywhere else until I could walk in.

After three weeks, my walking and standing still was not that great but there were improvements. I went from barely walking with the walker, to using it a little better daily. Even though I was not close to using it in public, I was using it around the house which was still a very unsteady and scary feeling. I asked for all the throw rugs to be removed from the floors after the fall; and after a few weeks I decided to give the okay to put them back.

At the end of four weeks of outpatient therapy, at three days a week, and working continuously at home, I was evaluated and granted another four weeks of therapy two days a week for forty-five minutes per session. The therapist informed me that due to my condition when I first came to therapy, she had given me an evaluation estimate of a four percent increase after the first four weeks but because of my determination and the extra work I put in at home, I showed an increase of eleven percent.

The first week of May 2009, my second month of outpatient therapy at the rehabilitation center began. During the therapy sessions, I still continued working at home. Most of my work at home was in the form of walking and trying to gain my balance for standing. I would place the walker in front of me while I watched TV, and at every commercial I would stand until the commercial went off. It became the longest three minutes of my life. Eventually, I started a five minute routine of standing with a fifteen minute break in between until my standing totaled thirty minutes worth of five minute routines. Even though I was getting a little better with standing, I still could not take a step without a lot of assistance and my terrible lean.

Weeks later, my standing time had increased from five minutes at a time to ten minutes. During this time, I realized part of my balancing problem was because the muscles in the bottom of my feet and my toes weren't reacting. It had never dawned on me before, the significant roll these muscles played in not only standing but also in walking. Just imagine trying to walk on a tight rope. I felt like a baby trying to walk for the first time because neither leg would cooperate.

In a matter of weeks, I started using a wide base quad cane in outpatient therapy. I immediately went and purchased one for practice at home. The cane cost $50, and I had bills to pay, but again I had to make the sacrifice.

I have to say it was the scariest feeling trying to make those two steps with the quad cane. The one thing the therapist would try to get me to do was to stop looking down at my feet while walking, but my feet would not move when I tried to walk while looking straight ahead.

Over the next two weeks, I went from eighteen feet to sixty-five feet of straight walking without a stop or sit down break, which was mostly due to my home routine. I was glad I was walking, but the walks were scary, tiresome, and unsteady. I had to take some weeks off from using G.I. Joe because even though I needed his assistance, I had bills that needed to be paid.

I used a section of the house from the kitchen to the back door which was a twenty-two feet walk. I felt safe in this area because the walls were close, plus there was a nearby counter top which gave me a safer feeling when I walked alone.

Before Memorial Day, my distance for walking at the rehabilitation center was seventy-five feet before I took a rest break. At the time, my doctor could not be reached for the approval of more therapy, but I continued my work at home for that week without going to therapy. I could do as much walking as I wanted in the narrow twenty foot space I had at home. By knowing the distance, I was able to monitor each walk, as long as

I knew when to rest.

Pretty soon, at home I was walking one hundred feet before stopping. I built my endurance up to where I could do four, one hundred feet walks in a day. In a matter of days, I increased it to two hundred feet, three times a day. Then one day after walking 200 feet straight, I felt okay and decided to see how much farther I could go. I walked another 200 feet without stopping!

Finally, after a week passed, the approval for a third month of therapy was granted. On my second day of the third month of therapy at St. Elizabeth Rehabilitation Center, the therapist and I, after putting the holding belt around my chest, started my normal walk around and back to the chair which was a seventy-five feet walk around.

Each time the therapist and I approached the chair; she asked me, "Are you okay?"

I answered, "Let's keep going." I must say, I did get tired but I got a second wind. On the fourth time around, I said to her, "Well like Kenny Rogers said, You have got to know when to hold 'em and know when to fold 'em, and I think I'm ready for that chair now."

When I sat down, she had a smile from ear to ear. I returned and amazed the therapist when I walked with the quad cane for a distance of three hundred feet without a pause or break. The therapist was so excited that she could not help telling the other therapists what had just happened. This was also an exhilarating feeling for me. It did my soul a lot of good to see a therapist so overjoyed about my accomplishments. If a stroke survivor experiences this from the therapist, it can inspire the survivor to strive to do even better. I had not seen this reaction from a therapist since 2003.

Even though I was able to walk for three hundred feet with the assistance of a quad cane and my therapist, I knew I had put only one drop in the bucket; but that was okay because I knew I had a long journey ahead. The end was certainly not close. I knew at this time I was making accomplishments but it was too soon to think that I had accomplished anything. I understood that I had to keep myself prepared for the long haul. I must walk a mile to gain an inch, which is what I used to say to my therapist. She asked me what I meant. I explained to her that I knew I had to put in a lot of work just to expect a little bit of progress, and eventually, the inches of progress would begin to show.

The month of June 2009 was my final month of outpatient rehabilitation. I have to thank the therapists at St. Elizabeth Rehabilitation Center for their continuous dedication and support. It really felt good to once again, be around medical professionals who were dedicated and who cared about their patients. I also wish to thank the therapists at St. Elizabeth Rehabilitation Center for restoring my confidence in the medical community. It did my heart a lot of good to know there are still medical professionals who show continuous dedication and support for their patients.

Chapter 10
Walk a Mile to Gain an Inch
The War Is Not Over Yet

My rehabilitation efforts went great. The only drawback was that I could not take two days off, because if I did my muscles would begin to weaken. During the three months of therapy at St. Elizabeth, I did get the opportunity to exercise, but having a forty-five minute session at two days per week, did not leave me with much time for exercise, and I did not have any exercise equipment at home. It had not dawned on me that plenty of exercise had been the missing link all the time.

Three months later, in September 2009; during a doctor's visit, my doctor saw how I was walking, which still required a great deal of effort on my part. He asked if I wanted more therapy and I agreed. At the same time I was supposed to set up the schedule for additional therapy, I realized I would only be subjected to the same routine of needing a ride to and from therapy. Kim would take me, but I wanted to lessen the burden already on her. Between her crazy working hours, taking Kaden to school every morning, and her own health problems to deal with, I did not need to, nor did I want to, add to her duties.

I already knew the routine about therapy. The first session of therapy would be an evaluation, followed by two days of therapy a week at forty-five minutes per day. On the fourth week there would be another evaluation and then I would be released from the program.

Although I felt the need for more therapy, the problems of going through the order of getting to the rehabilitation center and knowing what the outcome would be; made me have second thoughts. It did not make me want to give up; it just made me more determined, and I seriously began to think about what I needed to do. I decided to take matters into my own hands. I sat down at my computer, and for the next few weeks I began to jot down all the details of treatments I received from all the rehabilitation programs I had attended in the past six and a half years, including some of my own personal routines at the gym.

I went to work on putting together an exercise program that would gradually build up every muscle from the inside. I also included exercises for balance, walking, occupational, motor skills, and weight training.

Stronger muscles help support your joints and can give you more staying power when you are moving around. My in-home, self-made rehabilitation program included exercises to help build stronger muscles, which not only can help you regain your abilities, but it can also prevent stiffness and tightness from not being used. Beware that fluids can pool in your joints; so if you are not using or moving your joints it can cause swelling, pain, and skin problems.

Mobility can be accomplished but cannot be sustained without a permanent muscular structure built from the inside out. Realizing this, I began to look at all body muscles and the parts they would play if I planned to make a complete recovery. Years before, I had purchased inner muscle charts from some exercise equipment stores. I pulled out the charts, dusted them off and began studying them.

The first decision was to adopt the safety first strategy, so I called on my friend G. I. Joe again for assistance. I never want my friends or loved ones to not trust my work ethics. Accidents create distrust so whatever is done, do not take risks, and stay focused.

The only exercise equipment I had at home was a Health Ryder Rowing Machine and a couple of freestyle weights. This was not much, but I did not need much equipment to do what I had planned. I had G.I. Joe to take everything to a room located in the back of my house. Initially it was supposed to be my son's bedroom, but his dad was on a mission right now. That was my explanation to Kaden, who for such a young child, understood well because he wanted my health back also.

After coming up with the plan, I prepared my sessions like I was actually going to therapy. All exercises above the waist, or occupational therapy, were scheduled for thirty to forty-five minutes. The same times were set for exercises below the waist, or physical therapy.

As the weeks passed I decided to mix physical and occupational therapy within the same session. The reason I decided to do it this way was because of my experiences in therapy. Once a thirty or forty-five minute session is over in occupational or physical therapy, the second session can aggravate the first. By aggravating the muscles, it can make your therapy visit seem like a waste of time and accomplishments.

When I was doing outpatient therapy, after I finished with my physical therapy, I would have to go directly to occupational therapy. During occupational therapy, there would be a lot of sitting while working on upper body routines. Sitting would either stiffen or weaken my legs thereby making it harder for me to move around afterwards.

The transition was similar when I went to

occupational therapy first followed by physical therapy. During the walking and leg routines in physical therapy, the muscles in my arms would become aggravated.

In my new home routine, by combining the two in the same session, the down time from one session to the next was like a short rest period for those particular muscles involved. There would only be a few minutes of lapsed time between the upper and lower body workouts. This way, the muscles worked on in the previous session did not become idle long enough to become aggravated. It was as if I had given the muscle a five minute rest period. Also, while doing some exercises for occupational therapy, I started standing instead of sitting. This way the calves muscles, under foot muscles, trunk muscles and more; were all working at the same time I was working on hand and arm movements.

I had no prediction of my results, and I had no goals set. I had one saying when it came down to the work I had to do to gain improvement. *I'll walk a mile to gain an inch.* In other words, I was prepared to do a lot of work continuously without being concerned about immediate results. So with nothing to lose and not knowing what I would gain, I began to work on a schedule with a set of workout routines.

Once the muscle groups were identified and coordinated with my workout, then the amount of repetitions had to be decided upon. Too much exercise might discourage you from starting your routine, so I suggest that you always start off with a simple exercise regimen.

Next, when beginning a routine, never be ashamed or to proud to stop at a count of three repetitions. Finishing the entire routine and not being too fatigued to continue your normal day to day is important. You must not overstrain yourself, because building muscles from the inside out is a gradual but continuous process.

I color coded my workout routines by using the color green for over the waist or occupational exercises. Physical therapy or below the waist exercises were coded in blue, and the repetitions for each routine were coded in red. Most of this process was created from trial and error, and everything done each day was saved in my computer for future reference.

I set the start date of my workouts for January 1, 2010 for six and seven days per week. Each off day was scheduled when I got out of bed. My intent was to view everyday as an exercise day. This way my body would be the determining factor for each off day I took.

Needless to say, the next few weeks were exciting, yet also strenuous. I had each routine in front of me on the computer, so I would know what exercise came next. I tried to set a start time for each day, but if I did not start on time, I did not worry about it. My thoughts were to begin my routine whenever the time was right.

At the end of each week and sometime at the end of the day, I evaluated my exercises according to my needs and also to what my body was able to handle without becoming fatigued or too worn out before the next routine. *Remember, the reason for exercise is to build your body, not to kill your body.*

I changed my exercises on a daily basis if they proved to be too much or too little work. Some weeks, an entire exercise would be added or subtracted. Some weeks the number of repetitions were added or subtracted. Other times, exercises were temporarily removed and then scheduled to be brought back at a later date when my body was in better condition. Each week, exercise routines were stored in my computer for future reference, for keeping track of my progress, and as a reminder of the injuries from the strokes.

Because of muscle loss that can occur after a stroke, your body can become heavy and hard to control. Something as simple as leaning from a chair to pick up something or turning on a light can throw you helplessly to the floor.

From my own experiences, I realize the need and the benefits of long term exercise to build the body's muscle mass from the inside out. It is my belief because of personal experience that regardless of how much therapy you are given for occupational and physical therapy, if you do not build the required muscle(s) to a permanent position, you will need follow up therapy constantly because the muscle(s) will collapse in no time when not in use.

From the beginning my first priority was always safety first. In order to accomplish the *safety first rule* it is important to always have someone willing to assist and monitor your exercise activities.

I believe, because of my own experiences, that it can often be impossible to get government and private insurance providers to pay for long term services because of the pre-evaluation of a patient. This is how it works: There is an improvement chart made for every patient. Eventually the time will come when the evaluation percentage has been met or cannot be accomplished. The reasons could be because the patient's illness is too severe, or the patient has improved to a point of not needing as much therapy as before. Regardless of the reason, when and if this is determined, you will be released from the therapy program. I have learned that even after therapy, a stroke survivor still has a long way to go before even seventy percent of independence is achieved or regained. Being independent enough to handle life at home safely requires months of follow-up therapy.

No one can say exactly how long a stroke rehabilitation program should last. Each program is tailored to meet each stroke survivor's individual needs. A program can also change as your condition improves.

Generally, when someone has had a major stroke, there will be permanent changes; but with special exercises and lots of encouragement from family, friends, therapists and loved ones, some stroke survivors can relearn to do some of the things they lost because of having had the stroke.

Much to my surprise, by the end of April 2010, four month from after my start date, I was sitting in chairs with no arms, and picking things up from the floor without losing my balance. Instead of always leaning back in a chair, I now felt totally comfortable and safe sitting forward in any type of chair.

I was able to stand, reach around, grab, and pick up things, all with better stability and balance. I do not know the exact date when I reached this pinnacle. I only remember suddenly realizing one day that I was doing them. I never stopped to see what I could do. I just continued with my workouts.

Eventually, I had an exercise for virtually every part of the body, from my facial muscles to the muscles underneath my feet. I continued the exercises for six and seven days per week for one to one and a half hours per day. I was persistent, committed and dedicated to improving my health.

Now I am able to sit and lean forward in a backless chair for over an hour without strain. I can stand around for forty-five minutes and cook for two hours without having to sit. I can walk sometimes without touching anything for support for at least a hundred feet. I can walk with a wide bottom quad cane, not perfectly but well enough to move around a total of nine hundred feet at intervals of three hundred feet. I am able to safely take a shower without assistance in getting in and out of a tub shower.

Staying physically active can also be good for your mental and physical health. Know that while sitting in a chair or while lying on your back, you can raise your head and chest just slightly and work on your stomach muscles. While sitting in a chair, simply lean back as far as you can and use your stomach muscles to lean forward. In the beginning, you can grab the chair handle for assistance until you get stronger in your stomach. Eventually, you will be able to accomplish this without holding on to anything.

Increase the number of repetitions gradually. Just doing three to five repetitions at a time with a small break between will immediately show valuable improvement in your lifting in bed or reaching forward in a chair.

When most people see me today, they often greet me by asking me how I am doing. I used to respond by telling them that I was not doing well at all. Now my response is, "I've been better but I could be a whole lot worse." Having said that, I am determined to use what I have and work with it until I get the best I can out of it.

You must know that keeping a good attitude about

things, when you are feeling so bad, can help your progress. When you have a good attitude, you and others around you can deal with your condition much better, because while you are healing on the inside, others react to the way you look on the outside. When you show happiness, others are more likely to show happiness. If you show sadness, others are more likely to show sadness and pity for you. Let's face it, your true friends and loved ones are pleased to see you with a good attitude, and they often respond better because they probably understand that even though you are having a tough time, you try not to show it.

Did you know that a stroke affects not only the patient but family and friends as well? Changes in abilities may change how you relate to those closest to you. After a stroke, changes in roles and responsibilities may cause you, your spouse, or other family members to have feelings that make them uncomfortable. You should plan to talk about some of the emotions and feelings you and your loved ones might have after the stroke. These are natural feelings and emotions. Find people you are comfortable talking to about your feelings.

Each day when you get up, try to start your day with a meal because your body needs the nourishment. If and when you are in therapy, pay close attention to what occurs during your therapy session. *Remember this: The therapist is not only there to help and assist you in your recovery, but also to teach you what to do.*

When exercising, you do not have to severely work your muscles. Even if you can barely move the limb, you can attempt to move it. Just the strain of trying to move will help the muscle and also help the brain's connection to that muscle. This means that *doing a little something builds to a bigger something.* But also know that *a little of nothing builds a bigger nothing.*

After my last stroke in February 2009, when I started the first visit of outpatient therapy in April, I was in pretty bad shape. I was in need of a lot of help, but I came in with the attitude that I wanted them to help me but I also wanted them to teach me what to do once I went home.

On July 17, 2010 I walked at home without a cane a total of five times, and a total of three hundred and forty-five feet during a course of six hours. My rest periods were spent on the computer. The day before, I had walked without my quad cane for thirty-five feet, but my legs began to shake so badly that I did not have the courage to walk without the cane anymore for fear of falling.

Kim's mother, Cleo, also passed away on this same day, July 17. I decided to dedicate this day to her. Over a short period of time she had fifty percent of each of her legs amputated. In comparison with how I knew she must have been feeling on the inside, she never showed any feelings of discouragement on the outside. When she and I would talk on the phone, we would always talk about the motivation a person needs when dealing with life altering situations. "Strength inside is the key," she said.

Walking for me that day was very hard, but I challenged every step I made. This was not the way I had planned my day, but for some reason it seemed like the right thing to do. Each day from that point on was done the same way. Thanks to the loving memory of Cleo. God bless her and God rest her soul. I have to tell her, though she is no longer on this earth, "Thanks, Cleo for the talks we used to have. Thank you for the strength you left within me. I may not be able to explain it, but I felt it when it entered my body and my legs. I feel like I have been given a blessing today.

Week of July 27, 2010

I am walking nonstop one hundred feet, four times a day without my cane. I used the wall or a counter top to keep my balance and complete the distance when fatigue sets in.

I will continue this routine for at least six days per week with no set time to start or finish. The main objective of each day is to put the work in, and hopefully, one day it will pay off.

Week of August 2, 2010

I am now walking nonstop one hundred and twenty feet, four times a day without the cane. I continue to use the wall or nearby countertop to keep my balance.

I must inform you that I am not medically qualified in the capacity of a physician, nurse, therapist, or any person in the medical field. I make this statement of clarification because I never attended school or college for the knowledge that I have gained and that I am sharing with each of you. But there is an old saying that "experience is the best teacher". If this is indeed true, then I feel well qualified to share my knowledge and experiences about strokes. I have spent the last eight years of my life achieving, grieving, suffering, enduring, accepting, exercising, reading, self-motivating, consulting, advising, learning, coping, and hoping. I have lived what I am sharing with you. No medical degree can compare to the person who experiences firsthand the effects that a stroke survivor often goes through.

Week of August 25, 2010

I began thinking of things that I wanted to do, and I started to grow impatient. I began thinking that a year and a half had passed, and I still was not able to do a lot of what I wanted to do. Many times I would go to sleep only to wake up two hours later. I would try to map out a strategy for the next level of my recovery, but the next day I could not carry it out.

I had been walking so well inside the house that I wanted to get outside in the open space. This would create an entirely different challenge for me. At times I would get ready to walk outside, and the temperature would be in the mid to high ninety's. After several days and weeks, I began to reach points of not knowing what to do. I also knew that if I was to attempt to walk outside, I would need someone around. I called G.I. Joe and asked him to come over, but the temperature would be terribly hot and could be dangerous. I became so bored being in the house that I contacted my doctor and asked him to order more therapy for me. I was going to return to St. Elizabeth's Rehabilitation Center for the outpatient therapy, but I never set up a start date.

I lost more rest because I sat up night after night just thinking about the days in front of me and the days behind me, and wondering if there was more that I could do about my recovery?

Three weeks passed and I had not exercised. The strange thing about this was that even after not exercising for such a long period of time, I felt no weakness in any of the muscles in my body. This was very pleasing to know, because it proved that the work I had put in was paying off.

Eventually, I started to feel bothered by my family. There was turmoil and discord constantly brewing. I told myself that depression was settling in on me. One night I got out of bed and went to the computer. I decided to read over the draft of this book to check for errors. While reading it, I reached a point where I realized I was starting to feel better. The more I read, the better my personal thoughts became. I must confess I had begun to have doubts about finishing this book. But after that night, I know how fortunate I am to have something this powerful at my reach in a time of need, and that proves its usefulness.

I got up the next day with a smile on my face; and I felt like joking around. I did not have much money but I gave Kaden twenty dollars that evening for passing his test at school.

I started my exercise program and walking routine again. For some reason I felt like I was on a high again about my life and my recovery efforts. I felt like I had just gone out and purchased a new car or something.

I saw the doctor again in September 2010. During the visit I asked again to be scheduled for more therapy. I was progressing pretty well with my walking, but my left leg still would not flow like I wanted it to. I tried the treadmill but it was too exhausting. I retrieved my walker and began to use it again, and it seemed to work pretty good for me. I went outside and slowly began to feel safe walking alone with the aid of my walker.

I had plans to call St. Elizabeth's Rehabilitation Center to schedule the appointment for my therapy sessions, but those plans came to a sudden halt when I received a statement in the mail from Medicare. The statement showed the last bill they paid for the months of April and May of 2009. Medicare had paid $12,000 for my care. From May 1, 2009 to May 22, 2009 they had been billed for $5,615. This particular bill was for three weeks of therapy at three days per week for April and two days per week for May, and forty-five minutes per session, at two sessions per day.

I did not know how to react. I knew that it was not a bill that I had to pay but it was still disturbing. I also received the bill for the five weeks for inpatient care at Barnes Rehabilitation Institute. It was a total of five weeks, five days per week, averaging four hours of actual therapy treatment per day. The total: an astounding total of $31,000, which also included twenty-four hour daily care.

Before this statement arrived, I was ready for more therapy. But after learning the cost for my treatment, I could not get up enough drive to go through with it. After all, I had gained much more of my independence through my at-home exercise routine, all at no cost to Medicare or Medicaid.

I decided to begin my home exercise routine at full speed again. I also started a daily routine of walking with my walker. Even though I had begun to practice walking without my cane, I felt that walking with the walker created a better flow of natural movement in my legs.

At the end of the first week that I started up the exercise routine, I noticed that a more natural flow began developing in my left leg. I logged in five days of walking and a total for the week of 2,140 feet. I finished the week on Sunday with a total of 580 feet in two intervals. This day, all my walking was with a single cane only!

I broke my single walking record of 500 feet with a walk of 660 feet of straight walking before stopping. Thirty minutes later I walked another 200 feet nonstop. All of my walking was done with a mixture of my walker and a single-leg cane. The following day I walked a straight 400 feet, 500 feet and then 100 feet within a one hour period.

I began to notice that while moving around without any support at all, I gained more flow in my legs, more balance when I stepped or stood, and my sure footedness increased. Even though things were getting easier for me, I still keep my mind in the right direction. Whatever I am doing is working, but I was determined to increase the volume and continue my regimen.

October 20th through 22nd I achieved a single walking record of 800 feet, 850 feet and 1,000 feet. At the end of the week, I totaled 5,480 feet of walking, mostly with my walker but some was with my cane.

By the time I reached my 44th week of at-home exercising, I had made substantial progress. I kept my actual daily progress mostly to myself, but I had become so proud of myself and my accomplishments that I wanted to share my progress with someone, especially Kim. I was so eager to share my progress with her that one day I started telling her about everything. I talked nonstop but my excitement was short lived, and I wished that I had kept everything to myself. I guess I failed to realize that people have things going on in their life as well. Sometimes what we see as accomplishments may not be seen that way to others. After that realization, I started waiting until the house was empty, and I was all alone, before I started my routine.

My walking totaled 5,480 feet which was the most I

had ever done in a week. The good part was that my body still had energy at the end of the day. In the past, I could not do as much walking because later in the day I was struggling to get to the bathroom, or from room to room. I continued to use my walker to help increase my leg flow. I had made a decision that I would not start my cane routine until I was able to cover 4,000 feet in a week without being worn out.

When I do my walking routines inside, I use my single cane and it is beginning to feel better. Each day I am able to increase my distance.

Exercise Week; 48 November 2010

I started back on the treadmill. The work is hard but not as exhausting as when I tried to use it before. I have noticed a better feeling of stability in my legs. I feel more firmness and balance when walking. It feels like my feet are flat on the floor. At this time I do not know what is in store for me; but I feel the light beginning to shine a little brighter.

Chapter 11
A Need to Know and Nowhere to Go
To Stroke Survivors, Loved Ones and Friends

During my long period of recovery and getting my day to day life back together, I had numerous conversations with caregivers, loved ones, and friends of stroke survivors. I heard many stories of people who had simply given up and lost hope of ever getting better.

Some survivors who had gone through therapy were doing okay, but once they were in the comforts of home they accepted defeat. Some came home able to walk but fell one day and lost their courage or desire to attempt to walk again. The wheelchair became their safe haven. Some were moving around fairly well, but decided the work was too hard and their patience for quick results had just simply reached an end. Others decided it was easier to spend their days sitting and lying around being waited on.

One lady told me that her husband completed inpatient and outpatient therapy after his stroke. He was getting around on his cane pretty well but not perfect. After a while he settled into his big easy chair and his days and hours of resting and watching television became longer and more often. Eventually, his limbs became so weak he could not walk anymore. Now she says most of her husband's time is spent in the bed.

One day, a man who appeared to be in his late thirty's or early forty's approached me. After we talked for a while, he began telling me about his wife's stroke. He asked if he could have my phone number. He shared with me that after her stroke it had become hard to communicate with her. "She is sad every day and she hates being given any advice. She looks at life as if there is no hope and she very seldom has the energy to do anything. Luckily we do not have any kids to care for," he said. He wanted my telephone number because he wanted to see if I could talk to her. He was going to go home and tell her about me and hopefully she would agree to talk to me. Well, I never received his call.

I came to realize something. Whenever a stroke survivor talks to me about life after a stroke, I can relate a lot better to them, rather than someone who has not gone through it. Sometimes living with this illness can make the survivor feel as though they are in a dark hole; and the only ones to actually know or understand this feeling is another person that has been in that hole too.

A stroke survivor goes through many emotions during the course of each day. Many times we do not know where to turn for the real comfort we seek.

Often, you might feel like your comfort zone can never be reached because of so many unsure thoughts racing through your mind. One of the most critical thoughts is wondering if the person you share your thoughts with can relate to what you say. You, the stroke survivor, may start to believe that it is better if you safeguard your thoughts because sharing them with someone who does not understand is an injustice to all the emotions you harbor on the inside.

Chapter 12
Up Front and No Sugar Coating
The Truth Hurts But It Helps

During your recovery, instead of focusing on the bad, try to find some good that has come out of the situation. Try to put a little happiness into each day. Eventually, this will help in your desire to make progress toward your recovery. With that in mind, and as bad as you may feel, you must be aware that without the desire to get better, you will only slow your progress, and your condition may get worse. Without the desire to get better your loved ones, friends, medical staff and facilities, insurance providers and others will give up on you as well. If you are not trying, your loved ones and family might begin to wonder if coming home was the right choice for you. Friends will slowly begin to lessen their visits. The medical facility and insurance providers will more than likely recommend you to be admitted into a nursing facility.

You must know that the harder you try, the more independence you will gain. The more independence you gain, the better you will feel and the less effort it will be for your caregiver.

I am sorry for being so blunt at a time when emotions are sometimes at their lowest points, but hear me. When I had my second stroke on December 2, 2002, I was feeling the worse I had ever felt in my life. Pressure was on my body because of the muscle usage I had lost as a result of the stroke. To add to these horrifying after effects, I had a frozen face, a dead arm and leg, a crooked mouth, speech problem, and a rib cage that was squeezing the air from my lungs. I had no idea what the future held for me. One of the worse things I remember was all of the sugar coating. My feelings were all over the place. At times I felt strong enough to endure the unsteady feelings I was having, and other times I felt vulnerable and very sensitive. My expectations were high, and even though I wanted to hear something totally in my favor, I really wanted and needed the truth. I did not need anyone sugar coating the truth just to make me feel better. The truth was there to bring me down then conjure up the fighter inside of me. And believe me when I was face to face with odds against me, I came out fighting.

I may be alone in thinking this way at such a traumatic time, but I simply wanted the truth. What I needed and wanted to hear was someone to say, the verdict is not in yet on what abilities you will gain back after a stroke, but what we do know is if you continue to work and stay motivated, then chances are you could resume your life as it once was or close to it. With a stroke there comes only one for sure guarantee, and that is if you put nothing in, then you will get nothing out.

Know that, right now, you must work on putting aside the negative and focus on the positive. Do not look for an overnight cure, just look towards getting to work on making yourself better. Exercise is the key. Exercise will build muscles. Building muscles will build strength. Building strength is the key to recovery.

My aim for writing this book is to help people understand that physical activity will create a healthy life, and that a positive attitude can help you to overcome your disabilities. My aim is also to assist in broadening awareness of early warning signs of a stroke so you and many others can be better prepared to seek immediate help and very possibly reduce the debilitating effects of this illness.

I have visited hospitals and people's homes in an effort to encourage stroke survivors. I know very well the daily struggle it takes just to get out of bed. But I also know for myself that with determination it is possible for you to make your life better, even after having a stroke. I am not saying that everything will be like it was before you had the stroke, but to at least be able to stand on your feet once more and move around the house will be an amazing accomplishment. Getting from point A to point B can be pleasing enough.

From where I was after my third stroke on February 16, 2009 to my present condition I can say with boldness that if you remain confident, stay determined and exercise, the time will come when you too can reach into your kitchen cabinets again, and pull out those pots, pans and food, and prepare dinner for your family! I'm sure they will be pleased and surprised.

Next, concentrate on strengthening your arm, leg, and trunk muscles. By doing this, you can possibly put your wheelchair aside while you are at home. You can learn how to get around the house with your walker or cane or by simply grabbing and using furniture for support.

When you build these muscles, then in the event of a fall, you can increase the possibility of being able to lift yourself up on to all fours and crawl to a spot to grab a chair handle, a counter top or whatever is nearby for support to pull yourself up. In fact, do not wait on a fall; get down on the floor and practice getting up. Get someone to monitor you while you practice getting up into a chair or to a standing position. Practice using either leg first to figure which leg should come up first to support the lift from the other leg. Wear shoes that tighten firmly on your feet so in case of a fall you want lose your shoes. When moving around try to wear sure grip shoes, which will increase your chance of gripping the floor when attempting a lift. Also keep your knees flexible so they will bend more easily when positioning yourself for a lift.

Do not take risks. If you do fall, with enough strength built up, you could quite possibly find yourself able to control or slightly break your fall and lessen the impact and make your fall lighter. Do not get discouraged because of a fall, just figure out what caused it and be more careful the next time.

During my recovery efforts at home I tested myself by making short walks to the restroom or to where the television was located. Initially, I did not have a good balance at all, and sometimes I would fall. Most of the time I would actually see that the fall was not going to hurt so I fell knowing physically I would be all right. In the beginning, I would try to tell myself that falling did not bother me mentally, but it did because after each fall I stopped doing my short walks for a while. After a few days, sometimes a couple of weeks, I would soon build up enough inner courage and fortitude to try again. Like a person who falls off a horse, the more times it happened, the easier it became for me to get up, dust myself off and get back on.

I suggest when you are ready to start doing short walks, that you find an area in your house where there is a nearby wall, countertop, or dresser. You will find yourself being able to do more moving around independently than you ever imagined yourself doing. In an area where there is nothing to grab on, I leaned on the wall and placed my hand on the wall to walk, but I am still very careful. You should also be careful and cautious.

Eventually, try practicing carrying items in your hand, but nothing of great size or weight. The smallest object in your hand will enhance your cognitive skills. I started walking to the TV with a DVD movie to put in my DVD player. Other times, I would use a plastic bag from the grocery store, place food inside a Tupperware container and then put it inside the plastic bag, along with a bottle of water and carry it to the table.

The goal for me was to try to become as independent as possible without being careless. Do not look for assistance when it is not really necessary. When someone is around, they tend to try to be helpful with everything, which will get you accustomed to letting them. Do not accept help all the time, especially when you know you can do it yourself. Sometimes you should say, in a kind way, I'll do it, but thank you.

The simple process of getting to a standing position had to take plenty of maneuvering and adjusting. Just going to the kitchen for a glass of water was a major task. Sure, it would be easy to ask someone in the household to bring you a glass of water, but is this the way you want to do things for the remainder of your life? I don't think so.

My goal is to gain as much independence as possible. For me, accepting and looking for help on most things is not the way to achieve it.

My biggest challenge was getting in and out of the shower. This was challenging because I had to step over into the tub in order to take a shower. By having both legs affected by my last stroke, getting into the tub was ten times tougher than before. Before, the stroke had affected my left side only. Now my greatest problem was bringing my left leg up and into the tub without my right foot slipping. Even with the slip proof mat I had in the tub, I still had to be extra careful because when moisture settled on the mat, it caused it to have less traction. In the many times of getting in and out of the shower I called for help only two times. I have never fallen getting in or out of the tub/shower. When I am done showering, I do not know which made me feel better, accomplishing the task of getting in and out safely, or having had the shower itself.

The first thing you need to do when it comes to gaining your independence is to simply get up and move around. You do not need a lot of fancy equipment to start exercising, nor do you need to join a health club. Just put on a pair of comfortable shoes with good traction underneath and start walking. But, please remember not to engage in heart-straining exercises to reap big rewards.

Activities such as regular walking and moderate exercise can also help to lower your blood pressure. No other lifestyle change will provide such immediate and enduring benefits to your health and well-being.

If you have not been active for a while, start out easy with just ten minutes a day. Add five minutes a week to your walking regimen, building up to thirty minutes total, five days a week. Avoid strenuous exercise, especially if you are just starting on an exercise program. If you add some regular stretching or yoga exercises plus light weight training once or twice a week, you will have a total body conditioning regimen. Just make sure to be evaluated by a doctor or certified exercise specialist for your strength first.

One crucial aspect of regaining your health and independence is to overcome your anger and to manage your spirit.

As you begin your exercise program, you will want to look at your emotional and spiritual health. Does an unresolved conflict eat away at you? Are you often short-tempered with your spouse, children, or friends? Basically, repressed anger, frustration, and fear are hidden risk factors for depression. If you cannot manage it alone, or with friends or family members, you probably should consider therapy. There is too much at stake for you to risk losing the desire to work on gaining your independence.

If your depression goes on for too long without some type of professional input, you may not be able to pinpoint what is really going on, and your desire to improve your condition more than likely will begin to fade.

Chapter 13
About Strokes

___

There are two major types of strokes: ischemic stroke and hemorrhagic stroke. There are variations within both.

A third type of stroke, called a transient ischemic attack, or TIA. A TIA is a so-called pre-stroke, or a warning sign of an impending, serious stroke that could cause damage. A TIA is usually minor, generally does no damage, and is most often caused by a blood clot. It produces temporary stroke symptoms that then subside. But, a TIA is not to be ignored. You should get checked out immediately by your doctor or get to a hospital emergency department. Start immediately making changes to your lifestyle in an effort to prevent a more serious stroke.

Ischemic Stroke

Ischemic strokes are the most common. They make up about 83 percent of all strokes. An ischemic stroke occurs when a blood vessel becomes blocked, usually by a blood clot. Clots can form when blood vessels become clogged with fat and cholesterol. This condition is known as atherosclerosis.

In an ischemic stroke, blood is unable to reach the brain, and brain cells suffer from the lack of nutrients and oxygen that they would normally get.

There are actually two different types of ischemic stroke, depending on where the clots form. Clots that form *inside* a blocked blood vessel in the brain cause a thrombotic stroke.

Embolic strokes result from clots that form somewhere else in the body and travel toward the brain until the clot becomes lodged in a narrow artery, and causes a blockage.

Ischemic strokes may also be caused by a deformity in the valves of the heart or as a result of a condition called endocarditic. Endocarditic occurs when the lining inside the heart becomes inflamed. Clots form on these abnormal surfaces and later they travel and lodge in a small artery in the brain.

Hemorrhagic Stroke

A hemorrhagic stroke occurs when a blood vessel in the brain bursts or breaks, then causes bleeding in the brain.

Hemorrhagic strokes are most often traced back to high blood pressure. However, they may also be caused by an aneurysm. An aneurysm occurs when a weakened portion of a blood vessel balloons out, ruptures, and causes bleeding in the brain.

Another possible cause is an arteriovenous malformation, or AVM. AVM is when a group of malformed blood vessels rupture, and like an aneurysm causes bleeding in the brain.

Another cause of hemorrhagic strokes can be attributed to older individuals who have a buildup of a protein in the arteries called amyloid.

Although ischemic and hemorrhagic strokes occur differently, the risk factors and outcomes are quite similar.

People who are at greater risk for developing blood clots, including women who take birth control pills, are over age 35, and smoke, are at a greater risk of ischemic strokes.

Some health habits and conditions that increase the risk of bleeding in the brain; like drinking too much alcohol, abusing drugs, having a bleeding condition such as hemophilia or thrombocytopenia, or suffering a head injury may increase your risk of having a hemorrhagic stroke.

Furthermore, keep in mind that smoking, obesity, and poor diet, along with health conditions such as heart disease, diabetes, high blood pressure, and high cholesterol, all contribute to your overall stroke risk.

No matter how the damage to the brain occurs when a person has a stroke, without quick and proper treatment, the outcome may be the same. Understanding how strokes occur and how they can be prevented are important for everyone, but especially for those who are identified as being high risk.

For the first few days and weeks after a stroke, treatment is usually focused on preventing further illnesses and complications. Depending on what kind of stroke you had and how serious it is, you may be prescribed medications or given other procedures or surgeries. When your health condition is stable, rehabilitation professionals can assess your needs and refer you to the right rehabilitation programs.

After leaving the hospital, you should schedule regular follow-up appointments with your doctor and healthcare team to address your stroke risk factors, rehabilitation, caregiver support needs.

Most stroke survivors are able to return home and resume many of the activities they were involved in before the stroke. Leaving the hospital may seem scary at first because so many things may have changed. The hospital staff can help prepare you to move home or perhaps to another setting that can better meet your needs.

Frequently asked questions

Questions you may have about living at home after a stroke.

Can I live at home after stroke?
Going home poses few problems for people who have had a minor stroke and have few lingering effects. For those whose strokes were more severe, going home depends on these four factors:

• Ability to care for yourself.
Rehabilitation should be focused on daily activities.

• Ability to follow medical advice.
It's important to take medication as prescribed and follow medical advice.

• A caregiver.
Someone who is willing and able to help when needed should be available.

• Ability to move around and communicate.
If stroke survivors aren't independent in these areas, they may be at risk in an emergency or feel isolated.

How do I know if going home is the right choice? What changes do I need to make at home?
Living at home successfully also depends on how well your home can be adapted to meet your needs.

• Safety.
Take a good look around and eliminate anything that might be dangerous. This might be as simple as taking up throw rugs, testing the temperature of bath water or wearing rubber-soled shoes. Or it may be more involved, like installing handrails in your bathroom or other areas.

• Accessibility.
You need to be able to move freely within the house. Modifications can be as simple as rearranging the furniture or as involved as building a ramp.

• Independence.
Your home should be modified so you can be as independent as possible. Often this means adding adaptive equipment like grab bars or transfer benches.

Do you have questions for your doctor or nurse?
Take a few minutes to write your own questions for the next time you see your healthcare provider:

What living arrangement would you recommend for me? Is there a caregiver or stroke support group available in my community?
Your doctor may advise a move from the hospital to another type of facility that can meet your needs permanently or temporarily. It's important that the living place you choose is safe and supports your continued recovery. Your social worker and case manager at the hospital can give you information about alternatives that might work for you. Possibilities include:

• Nursing facility.

This can be a good option for someone who has ongoing medical problems.

• Skilled nursing facility.
This is for people who need medical attention, continued therapy and more care than a caregiver can provide at home.

• Intermediate care facility.
This is for people who don't have serious medical problems and can manage some level of self-care.

• Assisted living.
This is for people who can live somewhat independently but need some assistance with things like meals, medication and housekeeping.

Effects Of A Stroke;
The brain is an extremely complex organ that controls various body functions. If a stroke occurs and blood flow can't reach the region that controls a particular body function that part of the body won't work as it should.
If the stroke occurs toward the back of the brain, for instance, it's likely that some disability involving vision will result. The effects of a stroke depend primarily on the location of the obstruction and the extent of brain tissue affected.

<u>Right Brain</u>
The effects of a stroke depend on several factors, including the location of the obstruction and how much brain tissue is affected. However, because one side of the brain controls the opposite side of the body, a stroke

affecting one side will result in neurological complications on the side of the body it affects. For example, if the stroke occurs in the brain's right side, the left side of the body (and the right side of the face) will be affected, which could produce any or all of the following:

- Paralysis on the left side of the body
- Vision problems
- Quick, inquisitive behavioral style
- Memory loss

Left Brain
If the stroke occurs in the left side of the brain, the right side of the body will be affected, producing some or all of the following:

- Paralysis on the right side of the body
- Speech/language problems
- Slow, cautious behavioral style
- Memory loss

Brain Stem
When stroke occurs in the brain stem, depending on the severity of the injury, it can affect both sides of the body, and may leave someone in a 'locked-in' state. When a locked-in state occurs, the patient is generally unable to speak or achieve any movement below the neck.

What can you do to reduce your risk of stroke?
To reduce your risk of stroke, monitor your blood pressure, track your cholesterol level, stop smoking,

exercise regularly, and find out if you should be taking a drug to reduce blood clotting.

Is there any treatment for stroke?

Generally there are three treatment stages for stroke: prevention, therapy immediately after the stroke, and post-stroke rehabilitation. Therapies to prevent a first or recurrent stroke are based on treating an individual's underlying risk factors for stroke, such as high blood pressure, atrial fibrillation, and diabetes. Acute stroke therapies try to stop a stroke while it is happening by quickly dissolving the blood clot causing an ischemic stroke or by stopping the bleeding of a hemorrhagic stroke. Post-stroke rehabilitation helps individuals overcome disabilities that result from stroke damage. Medications and drugs are another treatment for stroke. The most popular classes of drugs used to prevent or treat stroke are antithrombotic (antiplatelet drugs and anticoagulants or "blood thinners") and thrombolytic.

What should a bystander do during a stroke?

During a stroke, bystanders should know the signs and act in time. If you believe someone is having a stroke -- if they lose the ability to speak, move an arm or leg on one side, or experience facial paralysis on one side -- call 911 immediately. Stroke is a medical emergency. Immediate stroke treatment may save someone's life and enhance his or her chances for successful rehabilitation and recovery.

Why can't some victims identify stroke symptoms?

Because stroke injures the brain, one is not able to perceive one's own problems correctly. To a bystander, the stroke patient may seem unaware or confused. A stroke victim's best chance is if someone around them recognizes the stroke and acts quickly.

Stroke Organizations:
American Stroke Association
This division of the American Heart Association offers support, information, and more.

National Stroke Association
The National Stroke Association devotes all its resources to stroke. Supported by major pharmaceutical and medical device makers, it offers information and support to patients, caregivers, and medical professionals.

Lastly, the more you know about strokes, the more chances you have to prevent a stroke. I wish you the very best in health.

Cle
A three-time stroke survivor

About the Author

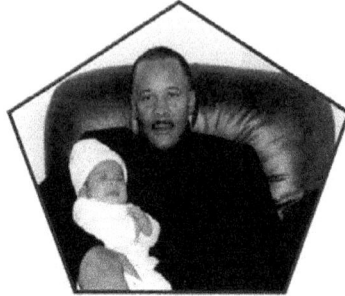

Cleothus Bell is a three time stroke survivor. He had his first stroke on June 6, 2002 at the age fifty-two. His second stroke was on December 2, 2002, and his third stroke was on February 16, 2009.

Nine years before his first stroke, he was employed as a demolition inspector for the city of East St. Louis, Illinois. He remained in this position for three years before he received a promotion to demolition director. After working as a demolition director for the city of East St. Louis, Illinois for a few years he moved on to work as the demolition coordinator for Saint Clair County until his second stroke occurred.

He has lived in East St. Louis, Illinois for his entire life. Because of the strokes, his former career is in the past. His future is living as a three-time stroke survivor.

Cleothus may not be medically qualified as far as having attended college from four to ten years and acquiring a degree that can be framed for the desk or wall; but since June 6, 2002, he has acquired three degrees - a *physical* degree, an *experience* degree, and an *emotional* degree. All have been framed to hang in his heart, mind and soul forever.

He has acquired these 'experience degrees' because of two hemorrhagic strokes, one embolic stroke, three different doctors, five different hospitals, two inpatient therapy treatment stays, three different outpatient treatment facilities, a private insurance provider and at present, Medicare and Medicaid insurance.

He has had the overwhelming experience of being paralyzed twice on the left side of his body. The first paralysis occurred during his first stroke on June 6, 2002, and the second time occurred during his second stroke on December 2, 2002. He had a six year recovery period before the onset of his third stroke on February 16, 2009, at which time he became paralyzed on both sides of his body.

Cleothus hopes by sharing his story, that it will help other stroke survivors, their families, their friends, medical personnel, medical facilities, and yes, hopefully, insurance providers.

Contact author for speaking engagements,
books, questions and reviews at:
bellcle@att.net

Book Order Form

Quantity	Description	Cost	Total
	Realities of a Stroke	$12.95 (each)	

BOOK SHIPPING INFORMATION
PRINT PLEASE

Name_____

Address_____

City_____

State/ Zip_____

Email _____

Phone (+ area code)_____

Money orders or cashier's checks only	Total
Subtotal	
S&H (add to total)	2.25
Taxes (If applicable)	
Total amount enclosed	

Make money orders and cashiers' checks
payable to Cleothus Bell
mail to
Cleothus Bell
P. O. Box 6323
East St. Louis, IL 62202

Thank You for Your Support

www.ingramcontent.com/pod-product-compliance
Lightning Source LLC
Chambersburg PA
CBHW060041210326
41520CB00009B/1221